TOOLS *for* STABILITY

A PATH TO PEACE OF MIND

MELVA FREEMAN

Copyright © 2021 by Melva Freeman

All rights reserved. No part of this publication may be reproduced, distributed, or transmitted in any form or by any means, including photocopying, recording, or other electronic or mechanical methods, without the prior written permission of the publisher, except in the case brief quotations embodied in critical reviews and other noncommercial uses permitted by copyright law.

ISBN: 978-1-953048-60-8 (Paperback)
        978-1-954341-63-0 (Hardcover)

 book are solely those of the author and do not necessarily reflect the views of the publisher, and the publisher hereby disclaims any responsibility for them.

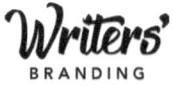

Writers' Branding
1800-608-6550
www.writersbranding.com
orders@writersbranding.com

Contents

Praises for the Book v
Introduction 1
Stress 13
Anger 44
Medical Help 67
Personal Experiences 99
In the World 112
Information List 123
Conclusion 129
Acknowledgments 139
About the Author 142

Praises for the Book

Reading the book *Tools for Stability* was a fascinating journey from another person's vantage point as they experience life with a condition many people have. *Tools for Stability* is a valuable teaching book for psychologist in training themselves and their clients, for people with family and friends that could gain a compassionate viewpoint which would lead to understanding what someone is going through. *Tools for Stability* will assist people going through a similar circumstance to know they are not alone. *Tools for Stability* opened me up to realize how close we all are to possibly shifting into another world from the one we may be experiencing this day. Melva tells a vulnerable story in an elegant and straightforward way. We can learn about people around us, people we experience in the grocery stores, common areas, family and friends, and gain more insight and show more kindness around this process to others. Reading Melva's book will no doubt be a useful professional psychology book. I believe strongly practitioners, hospitals, and universities could benefit from Melva's work. The book *Tools* is a positive book and perhaps life roadmap for people who are experiencing some similar situations. Melva herself shares a positive outcome in her own successful life letting others be aware they too can recover. Melva was courageous to write and share this book and did it so well.

Marilyn P.

I finished reading your book **Tools for Stability** about two months ago. It has made a difference in my life in a positive way and pieces of it keep coming back to me when I need them.

When you first asked me to read, it I was hesitant as I thought it was only for people who were diagnosed with manic depression. That would not apply to me. It is true I did get a greater understanding of what you, the author, deals with. I appreciate that. I also came to understand what we all had in common.

However, what was more important to me was a better understanding of what I had to deal with. I could use the common-sense and clear guidelines put forth in your **Tools for Stability**. One that stands out to me is, "All medications have side effects. Keep working with your doctor to find the best one for you." That really helped me when I was going through a rough patch with my eyes.

I especially like the sections on anger, dealing with family and friends, general health guidelines, and spirituality. Although I had heard them before they were organized and written in a simple, straightforward manner. I plan to reread them.

After I finished reading the **Tools for Stability**, I recommended it to a friend. She read it and has passed it on to other members in her family, both male and female of different ages. They have each found things that are helpful for them. Now I have a real problem. I don't have a book of my own.

I think it will be a valuable and helpful resource for a variety of people regardless of age, income or sex, i.e. families, individuals, ordinary day-today living, people in jail, people with medical issues, to name only a few.

Nancy

Just want to thank you so much for sharing your Tools for Stability with me. I shared it with my son and daughter-in-law and granddaughter. Don't know how much they read, but they said they found it helpful and more understanding than some of the books they have read. My daughter has read it. We both feel that your thoughts and advice are very easy to understand.

I have learned a lot by reading your book. I've come to have great respect for anyone with mental illness and to know the symptoms to look for. This both helps everyone, not just someone who has an illness. I have written some notes from your book.

To have been able to put your experience down for us to share has to have been difficult, but thank you for all of us who have so much to learn. May God continue to bless you, and may you continue to be a blessing to others.

Diane

I just wanted to thank you for writing this book from the perspective of one who had traveled the path of mental illness. You were so open with your struggles that I cannot help but believe that those who read it will be aware that you know whereof you speak. Great job!

Mark

Ms. Freeman exposes her experiences with bipolar disease very openly. Her recommendations for mental health are pragmatic and wide ranging. This is an excellent guide for people with mental health issues as well as their families.

Suzy

I met Melva at her work when I was needing assistance with my disability. I realized really fast that I needed to pay attention to what she had to say. She and I are almost exact opposites as people had personal interests and social lives, but inside we are kindred. We got through the same things and have had the same adversities. There was plenty in the book I already knew and plenty that I knew because I had lived it to. The best part though was the gems of insight and real-life fixes and advice that only someone who actually has similar problems can really know works. The experience in this book is immensely useful and it doesn't focus on being a victim or helpless but just how to recognize and work on the real-life struggles of being disabled. My favorite author is still Stephen King, but he doesn't write books that help me like this has. Thank you.

Marko

Beautiful pictures are developed from negatives in a dark room. So, if you see darkness in your life, be reassured that a beautiful picture is being prepared.

Facebook Friend

Introduction

The **Tools for Stability** has been a work in progress for many years. It started off as a workshop. As the workshop progressed and I added more to it, people kept saying I needed to write a book. So here is my book. I have learned a lot in recovering from bipolar I disorder, which is a mental illness, plus having PTSD. I wanted to share what I have learned because it will help anyone to have peace of mind. In telling my story, I am sharing my inner soul. Why? It is because I do not want you to have to go through the same things I have, whether you have a disability or not. If you learn one thing to help yourself, a family member, a friend, or a neighbor, it is worth it to me.

I learned about mental health versus mental illness. Thus, I changed this material to reflect what would help anyone, diagnosis or not. Take a look at the world around you. We all have mental health or mental illness in one way or another. When you are looking at the world's problems, think about it: people have had problems since time began. We hear more and see more about it because of modern communication.

If you looked at me, you would not know I have a mental diagnosis. I have what is called a hidden disability, like someone with diabetes or heart disease. I do not let it stop me from life. I work and take care of myself (including my finances). I cook, go to church, drive, have hobbies, pay taxes, travel, and vote. I have friends, read, live alone, etc. I work hard on my appearance. I have not always done that. Before, I am sure I looked like I was a mental patient. I was grubby and not always the cleanest I could have been. Now I make sure I have a shower and wear makeup. I no longer dress in jeans and T-shirts every day, although I still wear them.

You do not have to look far to realize our world is very troubled. Yet, that does not mean you cannot be have peace of mind. What would happen if everyone worked at having peace of mind? Then, if their families and their communities worked at having peace of mind, how much our world would be at peace? I challenge you to be at peace!

In my experience many people do not know the definition of bipolar. It is very hard to diagnose. My psychiatrist said,

> According to the DSM IV-TR there are four broad types of disorder. Bipolar I disorder is having one or more manic or mixed episodes. These are usually accompanied by major depressive episodes. Psychosis can be part of the manic phase; the mixed phase has both manic and depressive symptoms. Bipolar II disorder is one or more major depressive episodes. Plus at least one hypo-manic episode. Cyclothymia is another type. For at least two years, there are many periods with hypo-manic symptoms. They have periods of depressive symptoms. These symptoms do not meet criteria for a major depressive episode bipolar disorder. If

specified, in which the patient has features of bipolar disorder, but do not meet full criteria. An example would be very rapid alternation between manic symptoms and depressive symptoms. They meet symptom threshold criteria. Yet not minimal duration criteria for manic, hypo- manic, or major depressive episodes. Rapid cycling can occur with any type of bipolar disorder. The DSM IV-TR defines it as 'having 4 or more episodes in a twelve-month period.

According to psychiatrist Virginia Hofmann, MD, "We see patients who have rapid cycling. This happens over the course of hours or days." The **DSM-V** is the book that psychiatrists use to diagnose patients with mental illness. You can read the new **DSM-V** book if you want to find out how psychiatrists categorize mental illness. You can get it at the library.

In having bipolar I disorder, I have experienced psychosis. When I am in that state, it is like dreaming and sleepwalking. Sometimes I do not know what I am saying or doing but will say and do anything. Sometimes I remember what has happened, and sometimes I do not. Many times, when I do not remember what I have done in this state, I hear secondhand from family or friends. I have spent years of writing and rewriting the material for my *Tools for Stability* workshop. I rewrote it when I had changed and gotten better. Many people will find the information in my book helpful, even if they donot have a mental illness. My goal is to get this information out to as many people as possible. That way they can learn from my experience in a short time what has taken me twenty-five years to learn. I do not want people to suffer years like I did. Am I healed? For today, I can say I am in recovery.

It is embarrassing to have gotten manic, especially psychotic, and done the things I have done. So why, if it is so embarrassing, do I even share it with you? I share it for the people in jails or prisons, our biggest mental institutions. I share it with the general public so you will know what my brain does at this stage. It is something I cannot control any more than a person with diabetes can stop their diabetes. They can control it but not change the fact that they have it. I cannot change my brain, but I can take care of myself as best I can to keep from getting manic or depressed.

There are those people you know that you might think have peace of mind (some even commit suicide and people think they seemed so happy), yet do they feel at peace or look like they are happy? Are they in touch with their inner feelings, or are they hiding what is inside? If they are hiding their feelings, are they covering their feelings up with alcohol? Do they use drugs (prescription or street)? Or do they gamble, over eat, smoke, or do other addictive behaviors? Are you aware of your feelings? I was not when I started on my long journey. I used food to comfort me and could not be by myself because I was so uncomfortable in my own skin. Thus, I spent lots of time on the phone or I needed to be with people, whether they were mentally well or not.

Everyone has mood swings. Some have chemical imbalances or PTSD like me; hormonal irregularities; or diseases. Some people have a diagnosis of mental illness; and some, not. Mental illness is very common. Most people can improve their mental health whether they have a mental diagnosis or not. Working to improve your mental health, especially when you have a mental illness, is a lot of work. But it can improve if you work at it and have patience. Take baby steps to change the things you want to change in yourself and your life. You cannot change everything you want to in a day, but you can in your entire lifetime. Life is to enjoy. Make the best of it, and you will have great mental health.

Famous People with Mental Illness

One goal of mine is to erase the stigma of mental illness where the general public thinks a person can "Snap out of it!" or "Get over it!" or "Take your medication!" There are lots of famous people, past and present, who have had a mental diagnosis. As you look over the list of famous people with mental illness, think about voting. If you found out, before the election, that a candidate had a mental illness, would you vote for him or her? What contributions would our world have missed if they had not contributed what they did? Even if someone has a diagnosis, it does not mean they cannot contribute something great to our world. The following list is not complete, but it will give you an idea of what a person with a mental diagnosis can do. My list came from an unknown source. But if you Google "famous people with mental illness," you will find more. Many people listed have bipolar when we know bipolar was not known as a diagnosis at that time in history. It used to be called Manic Depression. I am sure these famous people were later found to have had a mental illness by looking at their writings or how they acted. If these people can do great things in spite of a mental illness, you can too!

US Presidents:

    John Adams - bipolar
    John Quincy Adams - depression
    James Madison - depression
    Franklin Pierce - depression, alcoholism
    Thomas Jefferson - social phobia
    Abraham Lincoln - depression
    Ulysses S. Grant - alcoholism, social phobia
    Rutherford B. Hayes - depression
    James Garfield - depression
    Theodore Roosevelt - bipolar
    Woodrow Wilson - anxiety, depression
    Herbert Hoover - depression
    Calvin Coolidge - social phobia, depression
    Dwight Eisenhower - depression
    Lyndon Johnson - bipolar

Other Famous People:

    Virginia Woolf (author) - bipolar
    Ludwig von Beethoven (composer) - bipolar
    Edgar Allan Poe (author) - bipolar

Vincent Van Gogh (artist) - bipolar
Sir Isaac Newton (scientist) - bipolar
Ernest Hemingway (author) - depression
Patty Duke (actress) - bipolar
Charles Dickens (author) - depression
Princess Diana (princess of England) - depression
Napoleon Bonaparte (emperor of France) - bipolar
Sir Winston Churchill (prime minister of England, Nobel Prize winner in Literature) - bipolar
Mel Gibson (actor) - bipolar
Michael Phelps (Olympic swimming gold medal winner) - attention deficit hyperactivity disorder

Tools for Stability

Too much stress + little to no sleep = mental distress, whether or not there is a mental illness diagnosis

Be the Solution, Not the Problem!

I once had a therapist say that I "chose to be mentally ill." I got mad at her, but I stuffed my feelings and did not say anything. That was my usual way of dealing with my anger at that time. After many years of teaching the *Tools for Stability* workshop, I finally got it. She was probably so frustrated with me because I had the "I can't" attitude. Below are some definitions of "choosing mental health versus mental illness." The first step is to recognize what is going on within and becoming aware of the problem. Are you a prisoner in your head or locked up in a prison or hospital?

Mentally Ill Definition = Depression

If you are staying in bed, will not take a shower or eat, isolating, and will not do anything anyone suggests; if you are refusing to take medication or refusing to work with your doctor to adjust it to make you feel better; if you are having suicidal thoughts and/or attempts, not seeking help; if you are complaining to people about how miserable you feel but you refuse to do anything about it, you are mentally ill. Some people attempt suicide, fail, and become more disabled than before. I worked with a man that shot himself between the eyes. He ended up blind! So, if you are feeling suicidal or even thinking about it, please get help! Believe me, suicide is painful for your family and friends. You can get help! It is easy to stay depressed and mentally ill, but it's a miserable way to exist!

Too much stress may be a source of the problem of mental illness. Some sources of the problem can be ***mentally ill definition = too much stress***: if you are too busy and not taking time for yourself. Do you have destructive anger? Do you use drugs or alcohol to keep going? Are you distracted and have dysfunctional relationships with others? Do you say yes, all the time (even though it affects your health and relationships)? Do you have no time to do fun things or relax? What about buying things to try to make yourself happy? Are your finances out of control? Are you under too much stress? If you know you are but you are not doing anything about it, you might be mentally ill. You can change your behavior to see if you feel better.

Some things that you can do to help your mental health if you have depression are the following: (1) try getting up, taking a shower, and eating; (2) spend a half hour in quiet time (including writing five things you are grateful for and one gift you have); (3) opening the curtains or installing LED lights to make it feel sunny inside; (4) play some music; (5) try getting out of the house and getting some exercise; (6) do a hobby or activity; (7) make yourself do something for someone else like baking cookies or pull weeds for a neighbor; (8) how about doing regular volunteer work or become employed? (9) call a friend, family member, or support group member; (10) get in touch with a therapist when you feel like you need someone to talk to about your mood; (11) if your doctor has put you on medication, make sure you take it as prescribed. Work with your doctor when you are not feeling well. You still might not feel great at the end of the day, but you will have done something with your life and done the best you could to improve your mental health. Working on your mental health when you do not feel good may feel like one of the hardest things you will have to do. You have to encourage and coerce yourself.

Mentally healthy definition = balancing stress. Be aware of your body and feelings by asking yourself, are you eating healthy meals, taking care of yourself mentally, physically, and spiritually? Have you uncluttered your environment and kept it that way, which in turn unclutters your brain? Are you making time for healthy relationships, fun, and relaxation?

Can you say yes to most of these questions? Are you taking steps to do something about the ones you say no to? Then you are working toward being mentally healthy. It might take time to feel better, but keep at it!

Stop!

Remember, it is nobody's fault that you have problems, an illness, or a disability. Everyone has something at some point in their lives. What is important is to live your life to the fullest, peacefully. You have to constantly tell yourself you are not your problem, illness, or your disability. Avoid complaining or introducing yourself as "I *am* disabled / I *am* mentally ill / I *have this or that* problem." Rather, say, "I am John (or Jane). I am an artist, volunteer, a community member, etc." You do not even need to explain your illness, disability, or problem unless it is required for some reason, for example, talking to Social Security regarding getting benefits. If you need to say you have a problem, illness, or disability for any reason, say, "I am John (or Jane). I *have* a disability."

If you are at peace, you can train and change yourself so you can be at peace, even if the entire world is falling apart around you. It takes practice, practice, and practice to change and take baby steps; but you can do it if you want to! Concentrate on the positive! What gifts and abilities do you have? Learn new things that can bring you joy.

Footprints in the Sand
(Mary Stevenson)
One night I dreamed a dream.
As I was walking along the beach with my Lord.
Across the dark sky flashed scenes from my life.
For each scene, I noticed two sets of footprints in
the sand, one belonging to me and one to my Lord.
After the last scene of my life flashed before me.
I looked back at the footprints in the sand. I
noticed that many times along the path of my
life, especially at the very lowest and saddest
times, there was only one set of footprints.

This really troubled me, so I asked the Lord about it. "Lord you said once I decided to follow you, You'd walk with me all the way.
But I noticed that during the saddest and most troublesome times of my life, there was only one set of footprints.
I don't understand why, when I needed You the most, You would leave me."
He whispered, "My precious child, I love you and will never leave you.
Never, ever, during your trials and testing's.
When you saw only one set of footprints, it was then I carried you."

I have added this poem because it helped me so much in my darkest hours, when I was having suicidal thoughts. I knew I would not follow through with my plans because I loved my family and friends too much to put them through that pain. In my reading of this poem, I added a line to help me in those dark hours: "There were times I was not able to see any footprints. In those instances, I knew I was being carried by the Lord, but I had my face covered in his shoulder crying, so I could not see the footprints."

I will explain about my faith later on, but this is just to let you know what has helped me. Please use only what helps you out of this book.

Stress

Another of my favorite poems is the following:

Don't Quit

(John Greenleaf Whittier, 1807–1892)
When things go wrong as they sometimes
will, When the road you're trudging seems
all up hill, When the funds are low and the
debts are high And you want to smile, but you
have to sigh, when care is pressing you down
a bit, Rest if you must, but don't you quit.
Life is strange with its twists and turns
As every one of us sometimes learns
And many a failure comes about When
he might have one had he stuck it out;
Don't give up though the pace seems
slow You may succeed with another blow:
Success is failure turned inside out
The silver tint of the clouds of doubt,
And you never can tell just how close you are,
It may be near when it seems so far; So,
stick to the fight when you're hardest hit
It's when things seem worst
that you must not quit.
For all the sad words of tongue or pen the
saddest are these: "It might have been!"
When care is pressing you down a bit, Rest,
if you must, but don't you quit.

Sleep

Sleep is the most important thing for your body to have good mental health. Pay attention to when you go to sleep. It should take no more than fifteen minutes to get to sleep. Keep track of the amount of sleep you get each night for a month or two to find out your normal sleep pattern. If you are having trouble with your sleep, try different things like having a regular bedtime, then getting up at the same time each morning, or not taking any naps or going to sleep when tired and getting up at the same time. Some people enjoy a nap, some cannot sleep at night if they have had a nap, and some might be groggy after a nap. Work hard on lowering your stress level. If you keep having trouble sleeping, talk to your doctor. You may need some medication, or you may have sleep apnea and need a CPAP machine at night. People are different and need different amounts of sleep to stay stable. If I am tired during the day, my body needs a nap. I can sleep anywhere from a half hour to two hours, feel rested, and still sleep my normal hours at night. Being too stressed causes many people not to sleep well at night. Thus, it is important to work at lowering your stress level as one of your first tasks to sleeping well. To find out how much sleep your body requires, see the paragraph on charting later in the book.

I have bouts of insomnia. The bubble technique (discussed later in the book) helps sometimes, but if I am really wound up, it does not work. One great solution I learned was to think about all the places I have lived starting from the first. Then I think of the things I learned or did there. It can put me to sleep very fast. However, if I am under too much stress I cannot get to sleep even if I do the bubble technique.

Stress

Having your stress level too high, whether from good stress (like planning a vacation) or bad stress (such as a difficult situation), can trigger symptoms, whether or not your medication works **or** even if you do not have a mental diagnosis. Balancing stress by having enough to **enjoy life** but not too much to be **overwhelmed** is extremely important for mental health.

One of the first signs of having too much stress is not sleeping well. Other signs are anger; holding your breath; a feeling of tightness in your body (e.g., neck tight, jaws clenched, or stomach tight); having headaches, backaches; getting distracted or anxious; or having relationship, job, or financial problems; etc.

I used to work at Disability Services & Legal Center for almost twenty years. For many years I worked with mentally and physically disabled clients. Most were homeless or near homeless with little to no money. I worked with people that needed housing. It was a really stressful job trying to find low income housing in a high rent area. The stress was so severe that at times I could not sleep well. I was repeatedly put in the hospital because I got manic. Each time I got manic I missed a month of work. What helped me in lowering my stress was to get a different position that was not so stressful. After years of working in housing I ended up dealing with paperwork, doing data entry, as well as staff training. I worked part-time, three days a week. I stopped getting manic. What a relief! I loved my job. Unfortunately, I was laid off of this job because they did away with my position due to lack of funds. I had to go on unemployment. I spent many months on unemployment hunting for a part-time administrative job. I went to Department of Rehabilitation which helps people with disabilities find work. I finally got a six-month training position at Petaluma People Services in an administration job. I enjoyed this work and hoped to get hired, but that did not happen. I was back on unemployment. Then I finally got a part-time position as a companion caregiver. This job is not stressful and I enjoy the people I work for. So far, I have stayed out of the hospital.

Ways to Control Stress

Some of the following suggestions are easier to do than the others. I will start with the easier ones.

Take a deep breath.

Breathing is critical when trying to reduce stress. The main way I can tell that I am under stress is if I can realize that my breathing is too slow or too fast. On occasion I have had to have other people tell me to **"Stop and**

breathe. " This has helped when I have been under too much stress or too manic.

Tell yourself, "HALT."

This acronym I learned in a twelve-step program. If you Google the acronym ***HALT***, there are many meanings. In this instance, it means, "Are you hungry?" "Have you eaten a nourishing meal in the last four hours?" "Are you angry?" "Are you lonely?" "Are you tired?" If you answer yes to any of these questions, do something about them and you will feel better.

Faith that your health and life will get better is critical.

Others have done it, you can too! ***You need to learn how and practice what you learn.*** Faith comes from wherever you get your spiritual energy. A spiritual base helps you get inside yourself. You can see how you are feeling. Do you want to change your life for the better? This is how you can be at peace in a world of conflict. Some people work hard to heal their lives; others stay angry for their entire lives. Some people cringe when you mention ***faith, spirituality, or God***. Has some religious institution hurt you? Ask yourself, "Am I willing to heal and enjoy life, or do I want to stay angry and miserable forever?" I am not saying you need to go to a religious institution to get better mental health. I am telling you that working on my inner spirit has helped me heal and get better mental health. It might help you also. I have had a hard time with a religious institution. But I have also changed and found a community that works for me, not against me. My community is very supportive as well as friendly. I have gained a lot from attending.

Have small attainable goals for each day.

Take baby steps to change the things you want to change in your life. You will go forward and backward, but *do not give up!*

Where you live can be very important. If you are living in a noisy neighborhood, consider using white noise or ocean sounds. Ask your neighbors to be quiet in a polite way, or consider ear plugs, or moving somewhere quiet. Another thing to consider is, are you being a noisy neighbor? If so, you should have your hearing checked. The most important asset for someone to have good mental health is to live in a good housing situation. If you cannot come home to a peaceful situation, how can you have peace of mind? If you are at war with yourself, how can you be at peace with your family? How about others you live with or your neighborhood or your community? If you cannot keep your house in order or clean, how can you help take care of our earth? If you cannot do all this or are unaware of how to have a peaceful life, how in the world can you live with peace of mind? How can we be at peace in our community or around the world? I know this can be difficult for many people. Even if you cannot change your living situation, there are many things you can do to change and have peace of mind. Be an example to others in changing yourself. It might take you years to change bad habits or situations. It has taken me a lifetime to change, and I am still changing. Changing will not happen overnight, but if you want to change, it is possible one step at a time.

Turn off the TV, computer, cell phones, and other electronic devices.

Ask yourself, "Do I have the TV, music, etc. on for background noise; or am I listening to it? Are these devices controlling my life? Am I isolating myself and not being around people face-to-face or getting outside?" If you answer yes to any of these questions, you are creating more stress in your head. This is not allowing your brain to be at peace. Notice what you are like when the electronic devices are off. Are you uncomfortable? If so, why?

Allow plenty of time for travel.

Arrive early for appointments and activities. Bring something to do when you get to your appointments. For instance, bring your favorite book, or sit and dream, or visit with other people (you might meet someone interesting), or people watch. This will avoid a lot of hurry. Plus, it will allow time for unforeseeable emergencies or traffic problems. When you wait until the last minute, you are creating stress for yourself. Plus, if you are driving, your driving may be a hazard to others.

If you notice you are not able to concentrate on what you are doing, especially while driving, ***stop, breathe, get outside and turn off any outside noise that you can until you can concentrate.***

Avoid purchasing, reading, listening to, and watching negative news from the media.

Remember the media plays on the negative. Think about how many times we have seen the 9/11 disaster or the Kennedy assassination. We do not need to hear about something that happened years ago. How many people have post-traumatic stress disorder from war? How many people are getting PTSD from watching the news? Is this triggering their fears or helping them have mental health? The majority of things happening in the world are positive. Search out the positive news. Do what you can to change the world to a positive situation. But remember, you cannot change anyone or anything, except yourself. Hold the media and politicians accountable! But do not let the negative media ruin your mental health and happiness.

Go for drives.

Do not drive when angry or manic or polluted with drugs or alcohol or in any way distracted. Get out in the country away from the busyness of the city. If you ride the bus, take the bus to the country for the day. If you are unable to do that, go to a park and experience nature. It will help to reenergize you and give your spirit a lift.

Know where your belongings are.

Put your possessions like your keys and wallet in the same place. That way you will know where they are at all times. Do not create last-minute stress while you are trying to race out the door.

Animals help, whether a real animal or a stuffed one to cuddle.

You might consider a pet to help you with your mental or physical disability. You can ask your doctor about having it certified as a service or companion animal. The law recently changed to where your service animal has to be dog trained to help you in some way. For example, if you have posttraumatic stress disorder, your dog might help you with your anxiety. If you have a physical disability, your service dog might help in picking up things off the floor. If you have a trained service dog, you can take it with you anywhere. That includes having it in your rental where the manager has a rule of no pets allowed. **But you must be able to clean up after your dog.** In my case, I have a betta fish named Manuel to keep me company. Even a fish can be a companion. If I wanted to, I could even buy a traveling bowl for him. Yes, they do make such a thing! But I choose to have him only at home.

Music is great for mental health, if you are listening to it and not having it for background noise.

When manic or overstressed, listen to calming, easy-to-listen-to music. Be careful with selecting your music; drums or horns might not be calming. When depressed, listen to fast, upbeat music. Pick some music from your favorite collection, something that will make you want to get up and dance or sing along.

Have some quiet time each day for at least a half hour.

This helps you get inside yourself to see how you are feeling. How do you want to change your life for the better, and how can you have peace of mind in a world of conflict? For your quiet time, make a space in your living environment. Make sure it is comfortable, or go out in nature. Pay attention to your breathing. When depressed, your breathing is very slow. You need to increase your breathing speed. When stressed, you hold your breath and your breathing is shallow so you need long, deep breaths. Meditation is very useful to help regulate your breathing. It can slow your thoughts and calm yourself. If you do not know how to meditate, you can learn. I had to learn to meditate, and it has helped me. Yet, when I am manic, my mind is racing so much that meditating is very difficult to do. During your quiet time, meditate or read spiritual literature. Self-help books or other inspirational books can help also. You can write in a journal, daydream, and listen to your inner thoughts. Say, write, or have affirmations posted around your house. One affirmation that helped me a lot I learned from a therapist. It was, "I am perfectly whole and complete." Others came from twelve-step programs that I have gone to. One is "One Day at a Time" or "One Minute at a Time," if things are very stressful.

Writing in a Journal

Writing in a journal can be most helpful for your mental health. It can also help strengthen your relationships. Choose a quiet location to get your thoughts out. Then destroy what you have written if you do not want anyone to see it. You can make a ceremony out of destroying what you have written. You can shred, burn, or find your own special way to destroy what you have written. It is beneficial sometimes to reread what you have written to see what your growth has been over time. If you do this, be sure to date your journal entries. One helpful technique for writing in your journal is to write a question with your dominant hand. Then answer with your nondominant hand. This uses both sides of your brain. Get out your anger in a journal instead of taking your anger out on others. Figuring out your part in the disagreement can be very helpful in relationships. Writing five to ten things you are grateful for can help relieve depression. If you live with someone that you are not getting along with, try doing a gratitude list. List things that this person does that you like. Each day include in a list at least one talent or skill or gift that you have as a way to boost your self-esteem. For example, can you wipe your own butt? Some people cannot. So, if you can, add that to your list. If you cannot, what can you do? I pasted in things that were special to me, like cards, or added encouraging quotes in my journals. Another thing that can be helpful is take a poem, like the "Don't Quit" poem, or other writing and expand on it. I have learned and gotten comfort from poems, pictures, and writing in journals. I found it helpful with my mental health progress. For twenty-one years, I wrote in my journals, filling two boxes. Sometimes, I wrote in the middle of the night pages and pages, not sleeping. Then I learned to do the cluster or bubble technique (see the chapter on anger), which does not take but a few minutes to do. I never read my journals like some people do. But I could not let them go, so I stored them in the garage, hoping no one would read them. I kept them in case someone in the future could learn something from reading them. Then I decided people are learning from this book; they do not need to read my journals. When I moved into my apartment, I decided not to take my mental illness into my new home. So, I tore them all up except the one that was not full. I did not read them as I quickly tore them up. But when I was tearing them over the trash can, I stopped when I came to a picture of my newborn grandson that I cared about. I figured this was God talking to me and stopping me. Many people will not believe that, but for me, it is true. In the last years, as my mental health improved, I lost the **need** to write. I have only written a few entries since I destroyed my journals. I do not know if it is because I have gotten better or that I moved to live by myself or my medication is working better, which helps me sleep. When I have been manic in the past, I have written volumes, as fast as I could write. I wrote compulsively in my manic state.

Laugh!

Have something that brings you joy each day. Having a good belly laugh or laughing so hard the tears come is the best thing. The greatest thing about the computer is laughing at e-mails or Facebook entries. I like watching comedy movies to make me laugh. It feels good to have a great belly laugh.

Unclutter your brain!

Keep a calendar for appointments and your to-do list for each day. By not cramming so much into a short period of time, you will have room for rest, relaxation, fun, and enjoying life. Include a short list of attainable goals for the day. List your appointments on your calendar, include phone numbers, in case you have to cancel. If you have trouble remembering your appointments, write a note to yourself and put it in a visible place, like your bathroom mirror. Color-coding entries on your calendar can also be helpful. One way to remember special dates is to put stickers on your calendar.

Organize your life!

Make your bed every day. This was a habit that took me years to do; but now, if my bed is not made, it bothers me. I took a time management class and learned it takes three weeks to make or break a habit. So, give yourself some time to make your new habits. Then start with your paperwork. Can you find your important paperwork in less than two minutes? If not, you are causing yourself more stress. If you are homeless, you can use an expanding folder to organize your paperwork. They even come in plastic and can be cheap at the dollar store or the $.99 store. Organize your kitchen or other spaces in your home so you know where things are. This will save time and stress looking for them. Have a place for everything, and keep it in its place. By having everything have its own place, you will be able to find things faster. This will save money, if you are in the habit of buying things that you already have but cannot find.

Are you feeling overwhelmed? Cut back on your activities. Take care of yourself, walk or do other exercise, read, or do something fun. Take a mental health day from work instead of waiting until you are so stressed you get sick. **Saying no** when you are feeling overwhelmed or overstressed is important. Think of it as if you had the flu. You would have to say no if you were sick. Taking care of yourself mentally is important. Practice saying "One day at a time" or "One minute at a time."

Gardening

Gardening is a great way to get out aggression and excess energy by digging in the dirt. It is calming to get out in nature and help things grow. You can even garden in apartments with house plants. There are many community gardens if you are unable to find some dirt to play in where you live. If you cannot find a garden to work in, call your local Parks and Recreation Department. They might have a community garden. You can even volunteer to start one. Help a senior who has property but can no longer garden, and share produce or flowers with them. Volunteer at a state park to help get rid of invasive plants. It is important not to overdo gardening so you avoid aches and pain.

> ***A hobby or job that you enjoy doing each week can bring joy to your life.***

Working as a volunteer or for pay keeps your mind off your illness or disability. It can also improve your self-esteem. Do you need a reasonable accommodation because of your disability? If so, you will need to tell your employer why. Otherwise, your employer does not need to know about your disability. My reasonable accommodation is working part-time. This helps me get my mind off my disability, plus gives me enough money to live on. Some people with a disability, whether physical or mental, can work full-time. It was very difficult for me to work part-time for many years. I felt so guilty as if I was "not good enough to work full time." When I mentioned it to my psychiatrist, he said, "Why ruin a good thing?" Since he said that, it helped me accept the fact that I cannot work full time like so many people can. So, I now consider myself semiretired. I plan on working as long as I am able. I know how bored I get staying home all the time, and that would not be good for my mental health. I was very fortunate that my past employer gave me earned time off that I could use for vacation or sick time. They also knew

I had bipolar. So, if I didn't sleep at night, I could call in, sometimes in the middle of the night. I let my supervisor know I would be coming in late or not at all.

The following are things you might need professional help with:

Are you trying to control someone else's life or the world? You can only change yourself! To change myself for the better, I cannot tell you how many times I said the Serenity Prayer over and over again. The "Letting Go" poem also helped me. To retrain my brain, I had a lot of help from therapists and twelve-step programs with this suggestion. Later on, I learned the bubble technique. Before my journey to wellness, I was an expert at trying to change everything and everyone in my life. At least I thought I was an expert. In reality I was very sick.

You have a fire hazard if your home is so full of stuff that you have a hard time walking around items! Is your home so cluttered there are walking paths between things? The clutter in your home or other environment represents the clutter in your brain. If your home is so cluttered, you may need specialized professional help. Extreme clutter is one sign of mental illness. There are self-help books to help in getting organized. If you uncluttered your home or other environment, you will feel much better. If you have a mental diagnosis, seeing the abrupt change can also increase your anxiety.

Do not try and do it all at one time. Set aside one to two hours, have a bag for trash, give away, and something to put in the things you want to keep. When trying to decide whether to get rid of something, ask yourself, "Have I used this or even looked at it in the last year?" If not, consider, "How important is it?" You might ask a trusted friend or family member to be with you, if you are still having trouble getting rid of things. When your time is up for the day, plan another time to unclutter and put it on your calendar. Reward yourself when you finish your task for the day by doing something for fun. Remember, "It is better to keep up than to catch up." It has taken me years to unclutter. My home used to be very cluttered. I am now down to a couple of boxes that need organizing. They are boxes of pictures and treasures from my ancestors that I want to put into albums. I want to unclutter them, but it is not a top priority right now, so I keep putting it off. I need to put a date on my calendar to get started with this project. But for now, they are under my bed and in my closet, so I do not see them often. Someday I will get around to them, but for now, they are not affecting my mental health.

Finances are a huge cause of symptoms (whether you earn a little or a lot). If you learn to live within your means, you will increase your mental health. Keep track of where you spend every penny for a month to see where you are wasting money. If you do not have much money, decide on your priorities and cut out all extras. Make a weekly menu, shopping list, and shop only once a week. Only go down aisles for the things you need that are on your list. If something is not on your list, do not buy it. Decide what is a need and what is a want? Are those chips more important than your rent? There are people living below the poverty line that live within their means and are happy. Then there are people that are making millions that have high debits and are miserable. *Money does not buy happiness or mental health. Having money problems can be another sign of a mental illness. So, it might be necessary to seek professional help.* I want to tell you my story about finances.

In 1990, my husband left me. He had taken care of all the finances during our marriage. I could not even remember how to balance a checkbook. I had taken a bookkeeping class in high school and finally remembered how to do my checkbook. I had a huge debt with legal bills, medical bills, and low income. I am grateful to my mom for helping me with my income for a few months and helping me with some major purchases. I was very lucky that some friends gave me a gift of a financial class and gave me books to read on finances. Since 1990 I have learned to increase my income by working part-time. Then I decreased my expenses by doing without the extras like cable TV. Finally, I live within my income and have a little to spare even though my income is low. Here are some tips I learned about getting out of debt: I had a large hospital bill that I could not afford to pay in full. When I got the bill, I immediately called the hospital. I made arrangements to pay fifty dollars each month. They agreed but kept sending me to collections even though I was paying my fifty dollars in full and by the due date. I kept accurate records saying whom I spoke with, when I sent my check, and what the balance should be. I also wrote down who said what. I found out one reason I was going back and forth to collections was because they lost five of my checks. I had to pay money to have the bank make copies of my checks and send them to the hospital to clear this up. I do not like being in debt, so I paid more than fifty dollars if I could. After the stress of this experience for two years, I found out that I was supposed to be paying 10 percent of the balance. I could not afford the 10 percent but still paid my fifty dollars. Luckily, I was not charged interest. One lesson I learned in all this was to keep a notebook that you cannot tear out the pages like you can in a spiral notebook. This is so if you had to go to court, the judge will be able to follow the steps taken. The most important things to keep track of is the date you contacted the agency. Write down the phone number or e-mail address. The name of the person you talked to is very important and who said what, how much you paid and the balance remaining. If you have trouble, you need to speak with a supervisor. Be assertive with the agency! Be accurate with your records, pay the agreed amount or more on time, and you will get out of debt. Recently, I started budgeting my money on an app called Every Dollar by Dave Ramsey. It is a free app and easy to use. I highly recommend using it.

Some Ways to Save Money

1. Set your thermostat for sixty-eight degrees during the daytime and fifty-five degrees at night.
2. If you are leaving the room for more than five minutes, turn off the lights.

3. Use a microwave as much as possible rather than the oven.
4. Lower your water heater temperature to 120 degrees or Low.
5. Is having cable TV a want or a need? If it is a need, switch to basic cable or no cable if it is a want.
6. When shopping, only go down the aisles where you need things. No window shopping, you might find things you want to have, not what you need.
7. Bring your own grocery bags; some stores charge for grocery bags.
8. Use senior discounts, if qualified and available.
9. Ask for a rain check if sale items are out of stock.
10. Brown bag your lunch instead of eating out.
11. Use plastic containers instead of baggies, plastic wrap, or foil.
12. When baking, use lids instead of foil.
13. Use metal utensils instead of plastic.
14. Make your own baby food.
15. Never grocery shop when hungry.
16. Never shop just to be shopping.
17. Plan your weekly shopping list, take it with you, and stick to it.
18. Grow your own food using seeds to start with instead of plants.
19. Buy in bulk food stores (with discretion, careful not to overspend); buy only what you need and have room to store.
20. Buy your clothes in the off season.

21. Do your own nails instead of paying someone else to do them.
22. Learn how to cut your kids' hair.
23. Buy washable clothing that does not have to be dry cleaned.
24. Wash and reuse plastic baggies.
25. Carpool or use public transportation instead of owning a car.
26. Put all your loose change in a jar; you will be amazed at how much it adds up. Use the money saved for special things like going to the movies or going out to eat.
27. Do your own car repairs and car maintenance, buying parts for your car at a junkyard. If you do not want to get dirty, learn about repairs so you will not get ripped off when having your car repaired or have a trusted person that is knowledgeable go with you when having your car repaired.
28. Shop around for auto-insurance discounts for multiple drivers, seniors, good driving records, etc.
29. Quit smoking, abusing alcohol, or drugs.
30. Buy store-brand items.
31. Form a babysitting co-op with friends and family.
32. Take a date for a walk along the beach or in the woods.
33. Make cards and gifts for family and friends.
34. Use discretion when using a debit card for purchases or use cash only.
35. Bicycle or walk to work or shopping.

36. If your income is low, file for earned income credit on your taxes.
37. If you pay for child care, make use of the dependent care tax credit or take advantage of your employer's dependent care flexible spending account.
38. Do not use the dishwasher dry cycle, open the door at night, and let them air dry. Only put soap in one compartment.
39. Shred old newspapers and use for cat litter.
40. Donate time instead of money to charities.
41. Make a compost pile from your leftover veggies if you have a garden.
42. If you use a credit card, stick to one card. Pay in full and on time each month to avoid charges. If you find you cannot pay each month in full and on time, tear up your card and cancel your account.
43. Instead of going out to eat, go for a picnic.
44. Use reusable wipes instead of paper towels.
45. Use cloth napkins instead of paper.
46. In the winter, if you have a ceiling fan, reverse your ceiling-fan motor so that the blades drive the warm air back down.
47. Close your drapes, blinds, and shades at night to help retain heat.
48. In hot weather, open your windows at night and close them in the morning to save air-conditioner costs.
49. Buy energy-efficient bulbs, or contact your power company about them; sometimes they are even free.

50. Save water by saving the water you usually waste while waiting for it to get hot. Use that water for plants, running your garbage disposal, washing machine, or drinking.
51. Call your water department to see if they have a water conservation program.
52. Wash clothes in cold water. About 90 percent of the energy used in a washing machine goes to water heating.
53. Make sure your dryer's outside vent is clean, and clean the filter after each load.
54. Use the Internet or phone book instead of directory assistance.
55. Drop unneeded phone services such as call forwarding, call waiting, or caller ID.
56. Shop around for long-distance and cell phone rates.
57. Use a "pay as you go" cell phone and purchase minutes without signing a contract.
58. Contact your phone company, and see if you qualify for their low income /disabled rates.
59. Use the library for books, movies, magazines, newspapers, etc.
60. Stay away from check-cashing places or borrowing money from people or credit cards.
61. Use coupons at the grocery store and try to shop on double-coupon days, if allowed. Only buy what you will use.
62. Buy fruits and vegetables that are in season.
63. Buy the store brand of food and drink.
64. Drink water or homemade ice tea instead of soda.

65. Drink tap water instead of buying bottled water. If you do not like the taste, consider purchasing a water-filter pitcher.
66. Shop for clothing and furniture at thrift shops.
67. Recycle!
68. Bring your own detergent to the Laundromat instead of buying it there.
69. Ask for generic prescription, when possible.
70. Use public transportation.
71. Exercise for free—walk, jog, bike to work, or get exercise videos from the library.
72. Move to a less expensive place to live.
73. Avoid using your ATM card at machines that charge a fee.
74. Get sample prescriptions from your doctor, when possible.
75. Shop around for the lowest banking fees or banks with no fees.
76. Cook from scratch avoiding processed or already-made meals.
77. Check your credit quarterly at 1-877-322-8228 or use Credit Karma.
78. Get a roommate to share expenses.
79. Shop at the $.99 or Dollar Tree stores.
80. Make your own coffee instead of going to a coffee shop.

For twenty-two years as an adult, I had roommates to help with expenses. The longest I lived with one roommate was eighteen years. Each time I got a new roommate or one left, I would add things to the following list. Many people have had bad experiences with a roommate. Or they have heard of someone else's bad experiences and are afraid to try living with someone. I encourage you to be brave and try it if you are having trouble with your budget in meeting all your expenses and if you have a spare room. It can be a pleasant experience. There are two key things to being in a good roommate situation: One is to respect each other. Respect someone's space and their faults as well as their opinions. It does not mean you have to have the same opinions, agree to disagree, if need be. It can be like meeting a new friend or family member. If you are a person that does not mind clutter, do not live with someone that is a neat freak. I can guarantee it will not be a pleasant experience. But it is still worth talking it over. You might have an agreement like my roommate and I did. We agreed that our bedrooms and bathrooms could be as messy as we liked them. But the common living areas had to be clean. The kitchen had to be cleaned after each use. If you try or have tried living with a roommate and it did not work out, give it another try. There is someone out there that could use a roommate too that you might be able to live with. You can use the skills you have learned in this book to help you. Remember, people change, as relationships change.

Suggestions for finding a compatible roommate:

If you decide to look for a roommate, give only your first name and meet at a neutral public location, such as coffee shop or the library, before you look at the room. This is for your safety. Make sure the owner of the property knows you would be renting before you rent a room. The person you are interviewing might be the owner of the property. Check with the tax assessor's office to make sure. Have the landlord put you on the lease agreement. If the property manager does not know you are renting with a roommate and finds out you have a roommate, you could both lose your housing. Pay your part of rent to the landlord, if you do not it might not get paid.

You might consider getting a credit report from the roommate, if you do not know the person well. Before you interview a potential roommate, make a decision on what is important to you. Answer the questions below. Then ask the potential roommate the same questions and see how many matches you have. This is a good way to see if you can be compatible roommates.

1. What is the rent/deposit? Is it within my budget?
2. Are utilities included?
3. Are kitchen facilities available?
4. Is the bathroom shared or private?
5. Do you want to live with a smoker?
6. Are you willing to live where drugs and alcohol are in use?
7. Is there a separate entrance?
8. Will you have use of the living areas of the house?
9. Can you have a private phone?
10. How do you feel about parties?
11. Can you have visitors?
12. Will there be overnight guests?

13. Will there be loud music? Can I play my music?
14. What about animals?
15. What about children?
16. Are there laundry facilities?
17. Is there a bus stop nearby?
18. What about parking for my car?
19. Close to shopping?
20. Is the room in town, or is it rural?
21. Who pays the bills?
22. Who does the cleaning?
23. Are you a night person or a day person?
24. Is there cable TV?
25. Do you want a platonic or sexual relationship? What about sexual partners visiting?
26. Who buys the food? Are the meals shared? Who does the cooking?
27. Get references.

Where to find a roommate:

You can check bulletin boards, websites, churches, Laundromats, and senior centers. Check the classifieds, social groups and organizations like churches, twelve-step programs. Advertise yourself on bulletin boards, pass out fliers, newspapers ads. Tell family, friends, neighbors, etc. you are looking for a roommate. Advertise on craigslist. Be cautious and make sure you meet in a neutral location, as I said before.

Just for Today
Author Unknown

Just for today I will try to live through this day only and not tackle my whole life problems all at once. I can do something for twelve hours that would appall me if I felt that I had to keep it up for a lifetime.

Just for today I will be happy. This assumes to be true what Abraham Lincoln said, the "Most folks are happy as they make up their minds to be."

Just for today I will adjust myself to what is and not try to adjust everything else to my own desires. I will take my "luck" as it comes and fit myself to it.

Just for today I will try to strengthen my mind. I will study. I will learn something useful. I will not be a mental loafer. I will read something that requires effort, thought, and concentration.

I received the below information from a support group a long time ago. The author is unknown. Whether it is factual is not known, but no matter, it helped me, especially when I was depressed.

Perspective

If you have food in the refrigerator, clothes on
your back, a roof overhead, and a place to sleep...
You are richer than 75 % of this world.

I received the following from one of my many therapists. To me, it reminds me of how I finally recognized when I was getting manic. It took me thirty years to recognize when I was getting manic. Then I contacted my doctor.

Autobiography in Five Chapters
(by Portia Nelson)

I
I walk down the street.
There is a deep hole in the sidewalk.
I fall in.
I am lost ...
I am hopeless. It isn't my fault.
It takes forever to find a way out.
II
I walk down the same street.
There is a deep hole in the sidewalk.
I pretend I don't see it.
I fall in again.
I can't believe I'm in the same place.
But it isn't my fault.
It still takes a long time to get out.

Tool for Stability: A Path to Peace of Mind

III
I walk down the same street.
There is a deep hole in the sidewalk.
I see it is there.
I still fall in ... it is a habit.
My eyes are open; I know where I am.
It is my fault,
I get out immediately.

IV
I walk down the same street.
There is a deep hole in the sidewalk. I walk around it.

V
I walk down a different street.

Anger

Our world is full of angry people. Are you one of them? Our prisons and mental institutions are also full of angry people. They can be inmates, guards, patients, visitors, or staff. What would our world be like if we all knew how and practiced how to deal with our anger in a healthy way? Would wars happen? Would family relationships be better, lowering the divorce rate? Would bullying stop in our schools and workplaces? Can you imagine peace happening because everyone knew how to deal with their anger in a healthy way?

Our prisons are our biggest mental institutions. Mental illness is not a crime, but we treat it as such. If inmates had proper treatment, instructions on how to get better, had encouragement, or if they did not have to fight the stigma of being locked up and/or have a mental diagnosis, many could return to society. They could be functioning people working and paying their own way. Instead of costing taxpayer dollars as they do now. If guards were more empathetic and caring, would it help the inmates? Many people, whether in the hospital, jail, or prison, do not have the knowledge about how to cope. Nor do they know how to change their situation. Our institutions do not use the latest and greatest medications. This is because the cost of some quality medications is horrendous. The other reason is that prisons do not have the time for the difficult job of finding the right medication. Most mental patients and inmates have to use medication combinations. It is difficult to find what medication works for each individual. This is because each person's body reacts different to medication. Many people do not understand that stress causes symptoms. These symptoms happen even when someone is on medication. The stress of being in jail, prison, or the hospital can cause symptoms. Also, not knowing the future release date can cause a lot of stress, which in turn causes symptoms. Many people after being in lock up, whether or not they are in the hospital, jail, prison, or are out with no place to go. Then because they have no other place to go, they are on the streets and become homeless for a long time.

I was lucky enough to tour the mental health unit of the Sonoma County jail. I was very impressed. That, to me, was almost an ideal jail. It was spotless, and the inmates looked well cared for. They had classes they could attend, if they were mentally healthy enough. There was artwork on the walls and a basketball hoop where they could get some exercise. Only one inmate at a time could play basketball. It was open to the sky, so the inmate could get some fresh air. There was a psychiatrist available at all times. They had caring and empathetic officers that had to apply for their jobs every year. The rate of return for inmates was very low compared to nationwide. I was very fortunate to present my Tools for Stability workshop to these officers. The one question they asked was how to deal with a violent inmate. I could not answer that question.

One time when I was getting out of the hospital, I was required to sign a paper that I would not own or have a gun for 5 years. This was as if I were a known felon. This law, I know, is to protect myself and others in case I become dangerous when I am manic, psychotic or depressed. This is to avoid hurting or killing someone. In the past, the only time I used a firearm was for target practice. I never owned one, although I had firearms in the house when I was growing up. This law is not practical because if I am manic or psychotic, I can get a gun from someone else. I can also use a butcher knife or bow and arrow. So, I do not see how signing the no-gun document makes me any safer around others or myself. My other reasoning against this law is that when a person is manic or psychotic, they do not have any control over their actions. Thus, they might not pay any attention to the law. When I am sane, I respect the law and will not have a gun in my possession.

The stigma of having a mental illness or being in lockup is huge. Thus, people are so embarrassed they do not want to get help or they are afraid of getting help. They might have also dealt with bad psychiatrists or medication complications. Sometimes they do not get treatment after they get out of jail, prison, or the hospital. They might not be able to get an immediate appointment with a psychiatrist. Or when they get out of an institution, they forget their appointment. Some do not have transportation. Often, their families or friends will not have anything to do with them anymore or cannot help. There needs to be someone to help them get to their appointments and get their medication. The stigma of having a mental diagnosis is huge. A person tries to avoid medication or seeing a psychiatrist. One of the main reasons I am writing this book is to erase the stigma. I have gotten better, with proper treatment. I have educated myself, advocated for myself, and had the willingness to change. I was so miserable that I wanted to change for the better. By trying several psychiatrists, medications, therapists, psychologists, twelve-step groups, I have gotten better. I have done spiritual readings, self-help books, and support groups. I have done writings to get things out of my head, and I began to change. My first therapist recommended I journal. I started in 1990, many times writing for hours. The main phrase I learned in twelve-step groups was to "Take what you like and leave the rest." I used this phrase often. This has helped me see what helped me when I was receiving so much information from all kinds of sources. I encourage you to use that phrase even when using the information in this book. What I find interesting is that as I got better, my writing in my journals slowed way down. Journaling has helped me more than anything, except medication. But I have had, at times, the support of my family and friends. I say "at times" because my family was not always available to help me, unless I was in the hospital.

I have had a great support system from some of my friends. Although I have lost friendships because of my illness, I do not blame anyone. I know it is difficult to be around someone when their symptoms are active.

The following, with a few exceptions, came to me one time when I was in a manic state. I wrote constantly, not even stopping to eat or sleep. I have changed a little of it to fit the Tools book, but basically, I have left it as is. This is to show you that even in a manic state, a person can do something creative. Many people like to stay in their manic state to create. I too like the manic state, but it puts me at risk of locked up, so I do not want to go there.

Destructive Anger Problems versus Constructive Anger Solutions

In choosing mental health, you need to have constructive anger solutions, not destructive anger. Twelve-step programs give the definition of insanity as "doing something the same way over and over again and expecting different results." Do you get your anger out the same way all the time and yet expect different results from other people?

Destructive anger can contribute to weak or broken relationships, hurt feelings, low self-esteem, insomnia, headaches, stomach aches, jaw aches, and other pains. Depression, high blood pressure, ulcer, heart attack, and stroke are also possible. Destructive anger leads to war and high divorce rates. Are you uncomfortable with the way you deal with anger? Are your relationships peaceful or troublesome? If they are troublesome, is there something you can change in your behavior to make things better? Remember, it takes two to tango, just like it takes two to ruin a relationship. What is your part? Are you willing to change to make a better relationship, if possible?

Anger is a natural emotion, but no one causes you to be angry. It is your reaction to what is going on in your life, what people are saying and doing, or what they do not say or do not do that causes you to be angry. There are some causes you can be aware of and work on and some you cannot do anything about. Maybe you just got up on the wrong side of the bed. Did you have a bad night's sleep or a bad dream? Triggers can be from a wide variety of reasons: too much stress, wanting to change another person or having someone trying to change you against your faith or values, world or political problems, frustration, impatience, PMS or living with someone with PMS, tiredness, being overwhelmed, trying to do everything and not saying no or delegating, perfectionism, feeling inadequate or helpless, having illness or disability or inadequate medical care, wanting to have complete control, feeling unworthy, in a hurry, unhappy with life, bored, lonely, grieving, not getting your needs met, jealousy, failing to accept you are wrong, being fed false promises, receiving mixed messages, attention-seeking, lack of security, excessive worry, fear, sadness, hunger, hurt, dishonesty, or residue from childhood.

These can all be harmful to yourself and/or others. In order to learn constructive anger solutions, you first need to know if you are currently using destructive anger. Some of the following may help you recognize yourself:

Destructive Anger

See if you fit any of the following categories. In my past, I have fit into all these categories. Now I practice constructive anger when I get angry. My life has changed so much now that I rarely get angry. I do not even have headaches or migraines anymore, which is a true blessing.

1. ***Rage*** is being way out of control, using verbal or physical abuse. It is sexual harassment, lewd comments, screaming, unable and unwilling to reason, terrorizing, throwing things, slamming doors, stomping, using vulgar gestures, swearing, belittling, unprovoked attacking, gossiping, bullying, threats,

blaming, sending nasty letters or e-mails, sarcasm, butting into someone else's business, intentional damage to property, sabotage, and road rage.

I will give you an example of my raging anger. This happened when my son was in preschool. He is now in his fifties. I had just cleaned his room, which I did not do often, because at that time in my life, I only cleaned when we were having company. After cleaning his room for hours, he left a pair of boots out of place. I screamed at him and threw one of the boots on the floor. It bounced up and hit the closet door so hard it put a hole in it. What would have happened if it had hit my son? I am sure he would have been hurt physically or emotionally. I had other raging moments, and at that time in my life, I was not a very good parent. However, I am lucky. Both my children turned out to be decent adults and parents. Although they do not know how to deal with their anger in a healthy way. Unfortunately, they are passing their destructive anger onto their children. My older two grandchildren have read my book and know how to have constructive anger, but as of today my children have not read the chapter of my book on anger. They have seen me manic and are afraid to read my book. That is because of the writing that I have done when I was manic that was so hurtful to them. Hopefully someday they will read my book.

2. ***Stuffing*** it can be a good thing (especially if your safety is in jeopardy) until you can figure out what to say or do. Sometimes, if your anger is stuffed long enough, it will hurt your health or relationships. It needs to be a fine balance. Stuffing anger can

contribute to feeling helpless or unworthy; being a doormat; being a victim; complaining; gossiping; holding grudges or resentments; denial of anger; avoidance of people or tasks; covering up by using drugs, alcohol, food, caffeine, and cigarettes; gambling; shopping; or any other addiction.

An example of stuffing my anger happened in my marriage, which lasted for twenty-three years. My husband had told me early in our relationship that if I got mad and yelled or belittled him, he would leave me. I was so afraid of him leaving I never got mad at him. However, I did gossip and complain, especially to my friends. I suffered migraines and other pain, was a doormat, and eventually did explode—so much so I ended up in the mental hospital. This was not a healthy relationship for either one of us, and it eventually ended in him asking for a divorce. However, I was so needy at the time that I was devastated. In looking back, it was the best thing that ever happened to both of us. I have not had a migraine since I got divorced.

3. **Passive aggression** is very hard on the person receiving the aggression to understand what the real issue is. It really does not promote constructive solutions. Some definitions of passive-aggressive behavior are giving the silent treatment, holding a grudge or resentment, destructive behavior, hostility, being forceful, refusal to cooperate, always having to be right, refusing to apologize when wrong, minding other people's business and trying to always fix their problems, people pleasing, turning anger toward self, being a martyr, pettiness, not willing to communicate,

ignoring concerns of others, giving mixed messages, selective hearing, nagging, and revenge.

In my passive-aggressive stage, I gave the silent treatment. Anyone could tell that I was mad by the expression on my face and my body language. I had to be right all the time and have my own way. I was very difficult to live with.

Sometimes it is difficult to take the time for anger resolution because it just is not the right time. Sometimes anger resolution takes days or months or years to work through completely. When you are somewhere you cannot express your anger appropriately, ***especially rage***, the best thing to do is to take a ***time out***. The world will wait. You will not be effective if in a rage anyway, so give yourself five to ten minutes to relax.

Thomas Jefferson said, "When angry, count to ten before you speak; if very angry, a hundred." When you feel so angry or the other person is so angry that you need to take a break, you can say, "I'm angry. I need a time out to cool down," or "You (or we both) seem to be angry. Why don't we take a five-minute break?" Then take a break, go for a walk or just get outside, breathe, calm down. While you are on your time out or walking, work on the following: (Using the bubble technique can be a great help in this process.)

A. Figure out what the problem is. **Is the reason you are angry because of one or more of the causes of anger (e.g., Are you tired, stressed, hungry, lonely, or some other reason)?**

B. **Whom can you talk to besides the person you are angry with?** This might be a trusted friend, family member, support group, twelve-step sponsor, or counselor. When picking someone to talk to, make sure they respect your confidentiality and not gossip or ridicule.

C. Brainstorm and problem solve and ask yourself these questions: **Can you do your solution now or later? How important is it? Is it doable? What are the consequences of taking the action you have come up with in your solution? Will you be safe?**

D. Set a course of action and do it, or let it go. If you cannot let it go, work through more of your anger using some of the suggestions below:

1. Go for a long walk alone or with a close, trusted friend or family member. This is not gossip time but working on your anger time. You might find someone who has been through a similar situation and see what he or she has done to resolve the problem. Think and talk about your anger. *What is your part? (Did you say or do something you wish you did not? Was what you said or did way out of line? Were you trying to control the person, their lives, or the situation?)* What you can do about it? What do you think might be the causes of their anger? Were they trying to control you? Are you being true to yourself and your values? What are your needs? What are the other person's needs? What do you have in common? Can you both get your needs met? Brainstorm solutions and/or compromises.

Tool for Stability: A Path to Peace of Mind

2. Write about your anger. Use the same questions as in number 1. Use your dominant hand to ask a question and your nondominant hand to answer. Do not worry about grammar, spelling, or being nice. Write about all the things you would really like to tell or do to the person you are angry with. Then burn or shred what you wrote. It is not something you want someone to find. Write to where you get your spiritual energy to ask for guidance.
3. Write a letter, **not e-mail**, to the person you are mad at, then mail it with a stamp **addressed to yourself** to cool yourself down and get some space. When you get the letter back, rewrite it. If you are still angry, do number 1 and number 2 above. Before you decide to mail it to the person you are mad at, have someone who is trustworthy like a twelve-step sponsor or counselor who will keep your ideas confidential, read it, and give you feedback. Think about what you would feel like or do if you got this letter. *Will it help or hurt the relationship? Ask yourself, Have I done everything I could to solve the problem? Will this disagreement matter in a hundred years? Is it really worth it to mail it? How important is it? What will the consequences be if you mail it?* If you decide not to mail it, shred or burn the letter. If it is worth it, go ahead and mail it to the person. They might be angry, but you have no control of their anger, and you did your best. Now let it go.

4. Make a box. Write about your anger, and put it in a box to let your spiritual energy (God, Higher Power, Spirit, Universe, or whatever you call your spiritual energy) deal with it.
5. Read a spiritual reading that fills your soul.
6. Get a gunnysack (from the feed store) and put dishes (from a thrift shop) inside and break the dishes with a hammer, then toss the gunnysack in the trash. This is only for people that insist on breaking things when they are angry.
7. Get a punching bag, punch a pillow, or use a plastic baseball bat and hit a chair. Punch and yell about your anger.
8. Knead some bread dough.
9. Run cool water over your wrists.
10. Meditate.
11. Say the Serenity Prayer that is used in twelve-step programs as a tool for a guide to problem-solving. "God, grant me the serenity to accept the things I cannot change." You can lead a horse to water, but you cannot make him drink. "The courage to change the things I can." Use strength and courage from wherever you get your spiritual energy. "And the wisdom to know the difference." You have choices: you can ignore the horse and hope he will drink the water (stuffing it), or you can force the horse to drink water (rage). The consequences will be that you hurt either the horse or yourself. The horse could throw up the water even if forced, you can break the horse's spirit, or the horse might

become afraid of you. You could shoot the horse and get it over with (rage), but it might be a really good horse and might get better. You might also be punished legally for your rage. Or you can lead the horse to water several times a day and sweet talk it into drinking water and let the horse make the decision if it wants to drink or not (appropriate). The consequences will be that he lives or dies, but you did your best to take care of yourself and to keep the horse's spirit vital. This applies to people too, not just to horses.

12. Have a good cry.
13. Do some cleaning of your physical space.
14. Go to therapy or talk to your spiritual director. Find a person that you can work with and respect. Go at least six weeks to see if you can work with them. If you cannot work with them, do not give up. Try someone else.
15. Go to a twelve-step program. Go to at least six meetings to see if it will help you. Get a trusted and experienced sponsor.
16. Go to a mediator.
17. Learn to compromise and agree to disagree.
18. Set healthy boundaries.
19. Draw or do other artwork about your anger.
20. Read or take a class on anger management or nonviolent communication.
21. Exercise.
22. Listen to music.
23. Tell your pet about your anger.

24. Garden or get out in nature.
25. Take a hot shower, bath, sauna, hot tub, or get a massage.
26. Dance.
27. Smash a bag of ice with a hammer.
28. Wrestle with a large "anger pillow."

If you decide to talk to the person you are angry with, after you have calmed down, you might communicate your anger by saying something like, "I became angry when.. I need..." and "I apologize for the way I expressed my anger. I wanted to say..."

After working through your anger, take action on the solutions you came up with. Do this only after answering all the questions that have been suggested. After you have done your best to work through your anger, let it go. Working through anger in a constructive way takes patience with yourself, as well as others. Work and practice, practice, and practice. **The calm will not come overnight.** Most people were not taught how to deal with anger to strengthen their lives and relationships, but you can learn, just like I did.

If you have trouble letting it go and your anger is still a problem, check out all you can on anger management on the Internet by typing in "anger management" in Google Search. If nothing helps, consider seeking professional help. **Don't let anger ruin your health, work, or your life!**

The way I deal with my anger now, which, as my life has gotten peaceful, does not happen very often, is to write about it in my journal. I use the cluster or bubble technique.

Then I talk to a trusted friend or the psychologists at my support group or my twelve-step sponsor. I work very hard to figure out what my part of the argument is and what I would like changed, if anything. For example, I was able to finally let go of all the anger I have had from being sexually molested as a child by a babysitter. I finally realized that he was just fourteen years old with raging hormones and an immature brain. After seeing him as an adult, I suspect he remembers, like I do. I have had nightmares since I was a child. Should I have PTSD as a diagnosis? Years ago, my therapist had me use the plastic bat on the chair to beat out my anger. I have also talked with experts on child molestation about what to do to get over it. I wrote in my journal for years. Then I wrote a letter of forgiveness to him. I finally felt compassion that he might be feeling guilty. I found his address online and his approximate age, which helped me. I talked to my twelve-step sponsor and read the letter to him to see if I should mail it. My sponsor recommended I **not** send it because it might hurt an innocent third party. I also talked about it in my support group. I ended up burning the letter at a park in the barbecue pit with my roommate as a witness. The amazing thing that happened was that after sixty years is my nightmares **stopped**! However, remember, this process took many years of work with lots of professional help and lots of work on my part. Just know it is possible to heal from past hurts.

How to Use the Cluster Technique

I learned the cluster technique (I like to call it the bubble technique.) in a journal therapy class taught by Kathleen Adams (**www.JournalTherapy.com**). I learned that this technique helps get the thoughts out of my head and onto paper so I can sleep. I found that this technique is the most important thing I have learned in my recovery! It helps me sleep, which keeps my symptoms down. I hope it will work for you too.

I want to describe my journal entry in detail. In the first edition of my book these pages came out blurry. Therefore, I'm leaving them out this time, but I hope you can get the idea of the cluster technique by my descriptions. You can also Google "Cluster Technique" and get a picture of several methods. The pages are from my journal on 2-4-09. You will have to use your imagination.

The drawing is like the spokes on a bicycle tire with bubbles placed along the spokes. In the center of the spokes is the word "worried." All the other bubbles, which are phrases or single words, lead back to the central word "worried." The words are what was going on in my head at the time and causing me not to sleep. This was the first time I used the bubble technique, and the first time I realized I was close to being manic. After using it, I was so excited that this technique had actually helped me sleep.

So now in your imagination, picture the "Racing Thoughts" page. In each quote represents a bubble. The center circle has "worried" written on it. Then there are lines going from the word "worried" to other bubbles

Tool for Stability: A Path to Peace of Mind

with words or phrases in them. The first bubble from the main word "worried" is "too busy." It has a line drawn to the word "me." Then the following bubbles with words or phrases in them. The first main bubble leading from "me" is "government." Then bubbles connecting to "economy," "negative news," "writing letters," "too much Internet news." They include "not relaxing," "work," "finances," "taxes," "pay or not," "manic or hypomanic?" "spirituality or manic?" "not sleeping," "too much stress," "racing thoughts," "physical problems." Each of these bubbles connect by line to the word "me."

The next major bubble that leads from "worried" is "coworker." It has a line drawn to the bubble "health problems." Next with a line from the word "worried" to the bubble is "brother." It has lines connecting to the bubbles with "what happens when Mom dies," "health," "cancer returns." In the next circle is "daughter" as the topic from the word "worried." The bubble next to it is "job insecurity," "my granddaughter," "no child support from Dad to Mom." The lines continue on to bubbles. With "marriage," "underemployed husband," "pregnant," "my grandson's graduation?" "bright," "wants to be a doctor," "won't do homework," "failing classes." Back to the main bubble from the word "worried" is "Mom." The lines connect to bubbles with "negative thoughts," "cancer or not." Then more bubbles and lines. Then attached to the bubble called Mom is "pain and suffering," "death?" "life?"

Next main bubble from the word "worried" is "son." It has lines to other bubbles that read "cancer or not," "life," "pain and suffering," "death?" "job," "health insurance?"

"wife and son," "unfinished house," "cannot afford," "left alone." That describes what was going on in my head that kept me from sleeping. At the bottom of the page, I wrote, "No wonder I've been awake since 3:00 a.m. with all these thoughts in my head. This is the road to mania. I have to stop it now!" I realized when I finished this page that I had no control of any of these topics. I could only control me.

The next page is "Serenity." This time the main bubble in the center has the sentence, "What can I do?" Then I did the same process as above.

At the bottom of this journal page, I wrote the following, "God is in charge of the other people and the world. I am in charge of me, and I can only change me with God's help. This is how I can sleep." Each journal entry page took me fifteen minutes instead of the hours it took be to write in my journal before I learned the cluster technique. I hope you get the picture of this technique.

After I did my bubble technique, I used the Self-Rating Mood Scale (see later on in the book). This is to check to see where I am on the scale. I use this scale to see if I need to contact my doctor and/or adjust my medication.

The Serenity Prayer helps me realize what is my problem and what is not my problem. What I have control over and what I do not. I learned this prayer in twelve-step programs. It has helped me a lot. If I am under a great deal of stress from things I cannot control, I have said the Serenity prayer over and over again:

"God grant me the serenity to accept the things I cannot change. The courage to change the things I can.

And the wisdom to know the difference."

I then read some pages from *The Language of Letting Go* by Melody Beattie, which is a tremendously helpful book.

Twelve Steps

1. We admitted we were powerless over alcohol—that our lives had become unmanageable.
2. Came to believe that a Power greater than ourselves could restore us to sanity.
3. Made a decision to turn our will and our lives over to the care of God as we understood Him.
4. Made a searching and fearless moral inventory of ourselves.
5. Admitted to God, to ourselves, and to another human being the exact nature of our wrongs.
6. Were entirely ready to have God remove all these defects of character.
7. Humbly asked Him to remove our shortcomings.
8. Made a list of all persons we had harmed and became willing to make amends to them all.
9. Made direct amends to such people wherever possible, except when to do so would injure them or others.
10. Continued to take personal inventory and when we were wrong promptly admitted it.
11. Sought through prayer and meditation to improve our conscious contact with God as we understood Him, praying only for knowledge of His will for us and the power to carry that out.

12. Having had a spiritual awakening as the result of these steps, we tried to carry this message to alcoholics, and to practice these principles in all our affairs.

Twelve Traditions

1. Our common welfare should come first; personal recovery depends upon AA unity.
2. For our group purpose there is but one ultimate authority—a loving God as He may express Himself in our group conscience. Our leaders are but trusted servants; they do not govern.
3. The only requirement for AA membership is a desire to stop drinking.
4. Each group should be autonomous except in matters affecting other groups or AA as a whole.
5. Each group has but one primary purpose—to carry its message to the alcoholic who still suffers.
6. An AA group ought never endorse, finance or lend the AA name to any related facility or outside enterprise, lest problems of money, property and prestige divert us from our primary purpose.
7. Every AA group ought to be fully self-supporting, declining outside contributions.
8. Alcoholics Anonymous should remain forever nonprofessional, but our service centers may employ special workers.
9. AA, as such, ought never be organized; but we may create service boards or committees directly responsible to those they serve.
10. Alcoholics Anonymous has no opinion on outside issues; hence, the AA name ought never be drawn into public controversy.

11. Our public relations policy is based on attraction rather than promotion; we need always maintain personal anonymity at the level of press, radio, TV and films.
12. Anonymity is the spiritual foundation of all our Traditions, ever reminding us to place principles before personalities.

*Copied from Alcoholics Anonymous Big Book

Note: *All twelve-step programs are based on the twelve steps and twelve traditions of Alcoholics Anonymous.*

Medical Help

My Story Part A

Most of my medical experience has to do with mental illness. What I have learned can help when dealing with any kind of doctor. It can also help with medication, hospitalization, or other institution. I want to explain about the lessons I have learned from the medical profession.

In 1987, at the age of thirty-nine, I was in the hospital, against my will, for the first time in a locked mental hospital. After that hospitalization, I had my first experience of visiting a psychiatrist. If I remember, I was on a lot of medication and did not talk, having my husband do all the talking. Yet he was not aware of what was going on in my head, so he could not tell the doctor what my symptoms were. After going through an MRI, CAT scan, and an EEG, I had my first diagnosis. My psychiatrist said, "Your diagnosis is right temporal lobe epilepsy. You do not need therapy, you do not need to come back, and your family doctor will regulate your medication."

A year later, after not sleeping and writing all the time, my husband took me back to the psychiatrist. This so-called medical professional actually shook his finger at me. Then he said, **"If you cannot stop writing like this, I will have to put you on lithium!"** I told my husband that I may need a psychiatrist, but I would not go back to that one. I never went back to him.

Years later I went on lithium, which caused many unacceptable side effects for the six years I was on it. Some people have great luck with lithium, but not me. It did not stop the compulsive writing, nor did it help me sleep. If it had, you would not be reading this book. Psychiatrist number 2 came two years later. This was when my teenage daughter was having so much trouble with me. She did not know who the real mom was, the sick one or the old one she knew. This psychiatrist sent me to a neurologist who said I did not have right temporal lobe epilepsy. He said all I wanted was peace in the world and in my family. He recommended individual and family therapy. Looking back, this neurologist was the only one with the correct diagnosis. Although I still need to take my medication to avoid the hospital. I do this because I have been psychotic before and do not want to get in that state again.

Psychiatrist number 2 did not believe in individual therapy. So, we went for family therapy. By this time, I was working full time. The psychiatrist took me off all my medication. This was after I saw the neurologist. The psychiatrist suggested that my husband and I have a date night, which was a total failure. At our third visit, the psychiatrist told my husband that he "could leave if he wanted to." This was because he was not cooperating. After that comment, I choose never to go back to that psychiatrist. As a result, my husband chose to leave after twenty-three years of marriage. Six months later my children also moved out, and I was alone for the first time in my life. My son was twenty, and my daughter was seventeen. My son moved out on his own, and my daughter moved in with her dad. I did not know my daughter was moving until the day she moved, which was the same day as my son. Needless to say, I was very troubled. I believed in long-term "until death do us part" marriage. I did not realize until many years later that I was much better off single. So, it was a true blessing for both of us that he did leave. Yet I am stronger because of what happened in our family. I was very dependent on my husband, and now I am a very independent woman.

In 1990 I was finally given the correct diagnosis of bipolar I by my family doctor. He referred me to psychiatrist number 3. This psychiatrist believed in over medication. He believed in the most medication for a year, then back it down to the least. I was still trying to work full time, but had tremendous side effects from the medication he had me on. This psychiatrist and my family doctor kept giving me more medication. This was to counteract the side effects I was having from the psych medications. They did this instead of taking me off the medications that caused the side effects. Having had the experience of over medication, I was through with psychiatrists. I relied on my family doctor for my medications. What I did not realize at the time was my family doctor should have sent me to another psychiatrist. This was because I have such difficulty with medication side effects. Remember not everyone has this much trouble with side effects.

I had two blessings from the many years of messy divorce proceedings. I had to go to many doctors ordered by the court. One was being required to see a psychiatrist for an evaluation. She told me I needed to get back to another psychiatrist and have my medication changed. At the time my family doctor was regulating my medication. The other blessing was from a judge who admonished me by telling me I needed to volunteer somewhere. He wanted me to go where I could finally get employed. I had been off work for five years at that time. I had the "I cannot" attitude and was volunteering at the Humane Society as a cat cuddler. I was terrified to work because I had learned that stress and lack of sleep caused my mania symptoms to appear. I was afraid of too much stress happening again. But I did as the judge told me to do. I volunteered and got hired for ten hours a month. For nineteen years, I worked three days a week. Even though I am not able to work full time any longer, it is a blessing to be stable and able to work part-time.

Psychiatrist number 4 finally took me off the medication that was causing me so much trouble (lithium). It took six years to get a doctor to take me off the medication that was causing so many side effects. Yet, when my adult children asked her if I would ever be back to the old person I was, she said, "No." Years later, I had a chance to meet her at a meeting for work. I told her I used to be her patient, which shocked her because I was doing so well and did not look like a mental patient.

Even though it took so long to get the proper medical help for me, do not worry! There are a lot more medical advances both in knowledge and medication than there used to be. It is possible to get help with education, perseverance, and advocacy. Some people can take one medication, and it works immediately for them. Others are like me and have to try different medication combinations. You might have to keep adjusting medications. This might be due to side effect problems, or medications not working. We are all guinea pigs. All medications, whether prescription or over the counter, have side effects. Even supplements have side effects. When taking anything, think of what the advantages are versus the disadvantages. Many people stop taking their medications for many reasons. Your doctor is prescribing medication for a purpose. I do not like taking or paying for my medication, but it is worth all the hardships I have had, especially if it keeps me out of the hospital and allows me to function enough to work and enjoy life.

My Story Part B

I have been very lucky that I have not been in jail or prison. Our jails and prisons are our biggest mental hospitals. They are full of people like me who have a mental diagnosis and have committed some crime when they were "out of it." As before stated in my book, if I'm "out of it," I do not always remember what I have done or said. I do not have any control when I am "out of it." Neither does anyone with a mental illness when they are "out of it."

Like a prisoner, I was not let out of the hospital until I was released by a psychiatrist and a judge that ruled, I could leave. (A judge and psychiatrist had to approve whether I was sane enough to be out in public, if I was in lockup past two days.) One time I was released from the hospital after a psychiatrist and a judge said I was sane enough. This was against the staff recommendation and my children's wishes. The judge and psychiatrist let me out of the hospital still manic and without any medication. I was back in the hospital again five days later because I was still manic. The second time the police came. I was not handcuffed like some people with mental illness are when they have to have the police involved. My family had the police take me to the emergency room. I was then taken by ambulance back to the hospital. This hospital experience cost me $4,000. Had the judge not let me out early, I would have stayed past the ten-day rule of my insurance company and not had to pay copayments. I had an attorney fight for me so I would not have to pay so much. We lost because the judge at the hospital did not keep records. So, I had to pay the $4,000. That took a long time to pay that bill due to my low income. But I paid it in full.

By good luck, my only jail experience has been visiting someone in jail for work purposes. I also visited a friend.

I want to tell you about a friend's experience with the jail system. I want you to know because it might do some good to change the system. Our prison system costs us big bucks and unnecessary time for inmates. It would help if they could be productive tax-paying citizens instead of inmates. Another reason I want you to know is because it could have been my experience. It could also be your experience or your friend or a family member.

The hardest part of my experience in dealing with the jail system was when my sixty-one-year-old friend was in jail. He was in the mental-health unit of the Main Adult Detention Facility, in Sonoma County, California. (I will call him George, which is not his real name). George went crazy because he got off his medication for a mental illness (paranoid schizophrenia). He was off for two and a half years without anyone knowing it while he tried alternative ways to heal himself.

What caused his breakdown, in my opinion, was the stress of having to move twice. This was after living sixteen years in the same place and living with the same person. After he moved, he lived alone for only the second time in his life. The only other time he had been in trouble with the police was as a teenager and that was a one-time thing.

In this incident, he was afraid of police brutality. George happens to be of a minority race. In the police records, it said that he threatened a neighbor and resisted arrest. He was afraid of the police. The police Tasered him and stood on his hand to handcuff him. As a result, they broke his finger. The Taser did not do anything to control him. George never received treatment for his finger because no one knew about it. Looking back, he feels that the police could have talked him down. He was scared, but they did not even try to talk to him. Why? Were these sheriff officers trained to deal with people with a mental breakdown? Some of the sheriff officers in Sonoma County have been trained, and some are not. Most police and sheriff officers do not get trained to deal with mental patients when they are in school. We are lucky in Sonoma County. NAMI (National Alliance for the Mentally Ill), people with mental disabilities and psychiatrists, have been training officers how to treat people with mental illness. It has been very successful but only if someone asks for a "CIT-trained officer" (Crisis Intervention Team).

George told me that he feels judges and police need to be locked up during their schooling. This is to have the experience of being a prisoner. I agree with him, yet for a true experience, the staff at the jail should not know who they are dealing with. Plus, I do not think the judges and police should know how long they will be there. They need to be frustrated. They need to have the experience of having to go to court as a prisoner. It would also be good for law enforcement officers and psychiatrists to be locked up in jails and hospitals during their training too.

For months George didn't even know where he was. He felt like he was a seven-year-old kid locked in a dark room while having to watch pictures of the Boogey-man.

George could only have visitors three days a week for about forty-five minutes while he was in jail. For being off his medication and having a mental breakdown, he was a felon for one year for resisting arrest. Even though he thought he was trying to protect himself from the police.

The other charges he received was a two-year misdemeanor for scaring his neighbor. George also had a one-year restraining order that he could not go within one hundred yards of his neighbor. His fine was $8,000 or $9,000. He cannot remember the total amount, but he was to pay for his neighbor's counseling and for her moving expenses. He still owes about $6,000. He can pay $25 per month due to his low income and his inability to work. George had three visits to his home (the first year) by the sheriff's department as part of his probation. They were looking for drugs and alcohol, besides making sure he was staying out of trouble. They dropped $1,000 from his required payments due to his good behavior.

When George had to go to court the first time, he was in chains. He had to wait in a small room on a bench. The chains were very uncomfortable. Somehow, he managed to get them off his arms. He later told the guard because he did not want to get into trouble. When he got to court, he was so upset he cried. The judge never talked to him the entire time he had court appearances.

George was in jail for five months until his friends posted bail. His friends spent approximately $21,000 in fees for his bail and a lawyer. George could have gotten a public defender, but his sister was very stressed out because it would take too long to get one. George's niece knew a lawyer, and since his friends had the money for these expenses, they were willing to pay. They also gave him money for incidentals while he was in jail. These incidentals were on a commissary list signed at night and put it under his door. The commissary list included snacks, little bitty packages of mayonnaise, and iced tea. It also listed shampoo, Top Ramen, pencil, paper, envelope, stamps, and phone card. He could order a pen, pencil, two-inch-long toothbrush, and soap. The dental floss was like a rubber band in a plastic container. Not everyone in jail had money. At least once a week, regardless of money, every inmate got a candy bar. If an inmate wanted a special book, he had to tell his visitor to order it from the publisher. The inmates could not have hardbound books, only paperback. George has curly thick hair, so he was not able to comb his hair with a comb from the commissary list. He looked like a wild man. George always liked to have a presentable appearance. Living like this and having to go to court looking like this was not good for his mental health. Usually, when he was struggling with his mental health, he still kept up his appearance. The only haircut he could get was to have his head shaved. George has always been picky about his hair, so having it shaved off was not an option for him. He could only get a shave with a dull electric razor. It was sprayed with disinfectant after someone used it. But that did not always happen. It took George half hour to shave because the razor was so dull. He had to try and sleep on hard three-inch-thick bed like a gym mat and a pillow about the same. He had a thin sheet, thin pillowcase, and two thin blankets. He did not get the sleep he needed. Can you imagine trying to live like this and get sane? Also, George complained about getting only two pairs of underwear a week. Sometimes the underwear was too big and did not stay up. He complained to the guard, but it did not do any good. In his state of mind, he had no idea when he was getting out. This was not good for his mental health.

Because of my experience in the hospital with few visitors, I could feel George's loneliness. It brought back painful memories for me of being in lockup. Having him in the jail made me realize what my hospital experiences had done to my family. Now I was on the other side of the fence. It made me realize their pain and frustration. I was upset with my friend for stopping his medication. Yet I am also grateful for him getting the care he was getting, even if he was in jail a long time. Due to my tour of this jail, I knew he was being well cared for, even though he did not think so at the time. He was away from society, so he could not hurt anyone or himself in his craziness.

I was afraid of what would happen to George because of the charges against him (felonies). I was grateful that he had so many family and friends that were helping and visiting him. I worried about his cat that was his constant companion and was mean to everyone else. Being mentally ill is hard enough; being in jail adds to the problems. Yet I can understand why some people in their mental illness have to be in jail. If they are violent and a threat to society, if they are very violent, they would be a threat to the staff at a mental hospital. The police get training and have the equipment (Taser guns) to protect themselves.

I want to talk about Taser guns. When I was on tour of the mental health side of the Sonoma County jail, I told the officer that was giving the tour that I did not approve of the Taser guns. He said without the Taser guns his officers would not have any protection. He pleaded with me not to take the Taser away from them. He said it was better than a real gun. At times all they had to do to calm an inmate was to point the Taser gun at them. They try their best not to use the Taser guns.

Hospital staff do not have the training and do not have the Taser guns to protect themselves as well as their patients. All they do when a patient is out of control is tackle them and force medicate them by giving them a shot of medication. They have the psychiatrist on staff to give approval. The mental health unit at Sonoma County jail has a psychiatrist on staff. But they have to have a judge approve of medication, which takes too much time.

George was fortunate that he had housing when he got home. His family helped him keep it. He was not homeless like a lot of inmates are when they get out of jail or prison.

Learning about George's jail experience, I hope has been helpful for you.

My wish is that you understand how a person that is insane needs to be in a hospital, not in a jail or prison! When inmates get out of jail but are not clean, shaved, and/or look like wild man, you will know why they look like that.

Charting Symptoms

Doing a monthly chart for your doctor will allow him or her to get valuable information about you. It allows your doctor to see in a brief moment what your month has been like. This is to see if you need medication or a change in medication.

A Personal Calendar is for people with bipolar or depression. This you can use to record many things. It is set up to record sleep, symptoms, stress, and medication. You can also record side effects, moods, and alcohol/drug usage. It is available free (if you order one at a time) from Depression Bipolar Support Alliance. They have a one-month calendar and a six-month calendar. You can reach them at **800-826-3632**. Since they are a nonprofit organization, it is nice to give a donation, if you are able. My doctor wishes all her patients would use the personal calendar. You can make your own chart for other illnesses. Any way you can, make a chart that will help your doctor know what your month has been like. Keeping a chart leaves time to talk with your doctor about other things that are important too.

Doctor's Visits

At your doctor's visit, it is important to be a self-advocate or have someone go with you who can advocate for you. Take a tape recorder, if you need to. If you go to a particular doctor, keep a small notebook for these visits. Have a list of symptoms, chart, questions, and concerns in order of priority. This will save precious time with your doctor. Keep a list of medications you have taken. List the dosages, side effects, what works and what does not. Ask your doctor if he or she want you to bring the list with you to each appointment. My doctor has the list of my medication on the computer in a handy place. Your doctor should work with you as partner. If your doctor will not work with you, you have the right to change doctors. It is important to educate yourself about your illness. You, not your doctor, should be in charge of your appointment and your body!

I want to give you some examples of being an advocate when talking to your doctor. When I was in the hospital in 2011, the psychiatrist had me on three different medications. This is common with bipolar. He tried to put me on a fourth medication. This was because one medication I took had a potential side effect of shaky hands. Years before this I had been on this medication when my hands were very shaky due to Lithium that I was on. The medication did not stop the shaking. When I was in the hospital, I kept refusing to take the medication for this side effect, because I did not have shaky hands. Even though I kept refusing this medication, it was in the little cup every time I had medication given to me. I am sure they did not put this pill back in the bottle after I refused to take it, which is a sign of wasted medical dollars. I kept telling the psychiatrist I did not want the medication. This fell on deaf ears. Another time while I was at the hospital in 2011, I took a liquid form of a medication I had been on since 2007. It was so sweet it made me nauseous. It also made me wonder if the capsule form I had been taking was a sugar pill. After I got out of the hospital, I wanted to get off the medication I was taking at the rate of seven pills per night. I worked with my psychiatrist and was then taking three per night. I respect my psychiatrist and believe her when she said if I take less, I risk getting manic again, which no one wants, including me. Years later, I was down to three pills per night. I have to have regular blood work done to track this medication. The blood test came out that I was not at therapeutic level. Thus, I worked with my doctor to get off this medication. I figured it was not doing me any good anyway. I also knew that if I got my sleep and stayed away from too much stress, I would not get manic. My psychiatrist requested that I e-mail her often to let her know how I was doing, which I do.

Another example of how I advocated for myself was also in the hospital in 2011. They had two psychiatrists on staff. I did not like the doctor I had. They had a chart on the wall that was for patient's rights. After I finally saw this chart, I remembered I could change doctors. I was afraid to try but decided I had to voice my opinion. They changed my doctor. It was that easy!

You should be able to talk to your doctor in an emergency. It might not be at the time you call, but your doctor should call you ASAP. There should be a covering doctor when yours is not available. I am very fortunate that I can email my doctors with nonurgent problems or questions. They e-mail me back within twenty-four hours, which has saved me a lot of money in doctor's visits. Plus, it saves them time to deal with patients with more urgent problems.

Medication

Most people have trouble with medication compliance at some time. If you do, ask yourself, "How is your life going without medication? Do you have a quality life where you are able to be active in your community? Do you live like you want and take care of yourself? Or are you miserable and in and out of the hospital or jail systems? Are you staying in bed all day or isolating? Are you where you want to be in life?" All medications have side effects. This includes prescription or over-the-counter medication, supplements, and even some herbal teas. What works for one person does not mean it will work for another. It depends on your body. Your doctor is giving you medication to help you lead a full life without hospitals, prisons, and jails. The pharmaceutical companies list all kinds of side effects. They do this to protect themselves from lawsuits. It does not mean you will have them. You need to consider the benefits over the side effects. What side effects are you willing to put up with to lead a full life? Weight gain for example is a side effect from many medications. This can be eliminated by watching your food intake.

    I want to give you an example of when I refused to take my medication. I was manic but not in the hospital. My psychiatrist put me on a medication that had a side effect of a deadly rash. He told me the medication did not work always for mania. I had been on the other three best medications for mania. Yet he wanted me to try it anyway to stay out of the hospital. I bought it, which cost me over $500, since I was in the Medicare doughnut hole. I had to pay 100 percent of my medication costs. When I got home, I read the literature that came with the medication. Then I called Medic Alert Foundation (you will read about that later) to let them know I was going to take it. That night I had it in my hand to take but got scared. I get rashes from using soaps or different textures of material. How was I to know if it was my medication causing the rash or something else? So, in my thinking at that time, I choose not to take it. As a result, I ended up in the hospital. After I got out of the hospital, I had an appointment with my psychiatrist. He told me I did not take it because I was unable to think due to the mania. It is easier to remember to take your medication if you have a weekly pillbox. They are available at any drugstore. Medication blood levels are necessary with some medications. This is to see the effects on the kidneys, liver, or thyroid. Ask a pharmacist or doctor about side effects before taking any medication. Your pharmacist or doctor can also give you a reliable website. This is to check out medication side effects. Check with your doctor or pharmacist to see if your new medication is compatible. It needs to go with what other medications or supplements you are taking. It is important that your supplements and over-the-counter medications go together. If you are having unacceptable side effects, ask to have something else. Say your doctor will not change medications due to unacceptable side effects. You have the right to change doctors. If you are on MediCal or Medicaid, it will be difficult to find another doctor, but not impossible. Keep the medication printout as long as you are taking the medication. If you have a side effect, first check the medication printout, then contact your doctor. If the side effect is not on the printout but you suspect it is from the medication, listen to your instincts, then call your doctor and the pharmaceutical company that made the medication. The pharmaceutical companies want to know for their research. They keep track of the number of people with certain side effects. Remember, they are scientists. They need your help too. Do not stop your medication all at once; always talk to your doctor first. Some medications can cause seizures or death if stopped all at once.

Besides all the side effects I have had, I had a doctor prescribe a diuretic when I was on Lithium. This was because my ankles were so swollen. I was very fortunate to have a good pharmacist at that time who said I could not take the diuretic with Lithium. He then contacted my doctor to find an alternative medication. Doctors are people who make mistakes, like everyone else. That is why it is so important to educate yourself about your diagnosis. Also educate yourself about your medications your doctor puts you on. In one experience I had with a medication I was given, I read the printout where it said I could not eat grapefruit. I mentioned it to my doctor, who was not aware of it. The pharmacist that I saw also did not mention it. It is important to read the print out for your own information and health. You might be a guinea pig, but do not be an **uneducated** guinea pig!

If you have a mental diagnosis that requires medication, are you taking it as prescribed? Are you working with your doctor for your body and wellness? Many people with a mental diagnosis decide they feel okay, so they stop taking their medication. When I talk to people like this, I tell them they have two options: (1) Take their medication as prescribed while working with their doctor, even if they have unacceptable side effects. (2) Don't take their medication as prescribed and end up in the hospital, prison, or jail. If you end up in the hospital, prison, or jail the staff can force medicate you. It is your choice. I urge you to think the worst-case scenarios. Many people have problems with medication side effects. Some doctors refuse to change the medication. Remember, if that is your situation you have the option to change doctors. Before you stop taking your medication, think about it. Say your medications that you are taking for Diabetes or heart problems were working. Would you stop taking them? I do not think so. So, think about it before you stop taking your psychiatric medication.

Medic Alert Foundation

Medic Alert Foundation, 800-432-5378, is a nonprofit organization. They have emergency bracelets, necklaces, and watches. They are in business to help emergency-response personnel. If you are unconscious, the emergency people can contact Medic Alert. They can then know your medical information and can contact your family or friend. This is important if you are on any medication or have any allergies. You want the emergency people to know what medication you are on to avoid complications. Help with the cost is available if you request and qualify for it. Medic Alert is nonprofit, so donations help.

I have had a Medic Alert bracelet for years. It has my member number, their 800 number, and my allergies written on my bracelet. If I am unconscious and the emergency personnel call the 800 number, they can get a list of the medications, and dosages that I am on. They even know what time of day I take the medication. They have a list of emergency contact numbers, like those of my doctors and my family contacts.

Medic Alert Foundation charges an annual fee. But it is free if you make any changes to your account during the year. I do not take any medication before I notify Medic Alert. I do this because I have had so many side effects. I want to make sure any emergency personnel have the latest in my medications. This is in case there is a problem with the new medication.

Eat Well

If you are having any health problems, look at what is in your food. Can you understand what is on the label? If not, it is not helping your health. Are you eating a lot of fast food or junk food? In the long run, that affects your health. Are you an emotional eater or food addict? If you are an emotional eater or food addict, there are twelve-step programs to help you (Food Addicts Anonymous and Overeaters Anonymous). This works even if your medication causes weight gain. I learned from Dr. Phil, "It isn't the medication that causes weight gain. It is the food you put in your mouth." When I heard him say that several years ago, I weighed 217 pounds, which was my highest weight. I worked hard but got my weight down to 155 pounds by going to Food Addicts Anonymous and not eating sugar or flour. (I am six-foot-tall with small bones, so that is a good weight for me.) Today I weigh 190 pounds. That is because I ate flour and sugar when I was in the hospital in 2011 and have not been careful with what I eat since then. Currently, I attend TOPS (Take Off Pounds Sensibly). I am working on it. One of my medications causes weight gain, which makes it harder to lose weight. I know I will get rid of the extra pounds if I keep at it. I have supportive friends in TOPS.

Avoid

If you use alcohol, drugs, nicotine, and caffeine they will affect your moods. Caffeine is in coffee, chocolate, some tea, and sodas. Using these products counteracts what your doctor is trying to do with your medication. If you are abusing drugs or alcohol, then someone else says you have a problem, ask yourself, "Am I an alcoholic, a drug addict, or mentally ill?" The following definition was by a doctor at a workshop held in Santa Rosa. I do not remember his name, but I remember his message: ***"If you use drugs or alcohol to get high, you are an addict. If you use drugs or alcohol to feel better you are mentally ill. If you use drugs or alcohol to get high and to feel better, you are a mentally ill addict."*** No matter what, you can change if you want to put the work into changing.

Exercise

Exercise is one of the greatest tools to increase your mental as well as physical health. It changes your brain chemistry. Make sure you discuss with your doctor before starting an exercise program. Walking is cheap, if you are able to do it. Moving as fast as you are able, when you need to, to get excess energy out or as a stress relief is a great benefit. If you have a lot of aches and pains and are unable to walk, consider water therapy or sitting and wiggling or moving. Climbing the stairs or parking at the back of the parking lot are great ways to get in exercise. I live on the third floor and use the stairs as much as I can. Sometimes I walk the halls of my apartment building including seven stairwells. Check with your medical insurance company; some companies give you free gym membership. This can be especially true if you are a senior. Only do as much exercise as you are able to. If you hurt, ***stop***!

Therapy or Psychologist

If you are doing all you can to improve your relationships and your mental health but you are still having difficulty, consider seeing a therapist or psychologist to help you. Make sure you get one you can work with and learn from. The person you choose should be supportive but also someone who will encourage you to grow to be the best person you can be. Many will work with you on a sliding scale.

Friends and Family

Friends and family can be a support or a hindrance to recovery. If yours are a hindrance, ask yourself, "Do I need to learn to set boundaries so I can put up with the relationship?" or "What can I change in myself to make the relationship stronger, if possible?" or "Have I sought professional help and guidance?" or "Do I need to stay away from them for a while for my mental health?" Try making a gratitude list of the things that are good about this person.

Make a pro and con list of what it will be like if you keep or end the relationship. If after a while nothing changes and you have tried everything, for your own health, you need to consider ending the relationship. This can be very difficult! You need to ask, "What are my priorities, my health or an unhealthy relationship that is making me ill?" ***Remember it is your life!***

I have been on both ends of friendship and family issues. I keep friends a long time, yet I have lost some friends because they cannot be around my illness any longer. This has been very painful at times, but I understand. I have learned in twelve-step programs and therapy how to set healthy boundaries, where before I would let people walk all over me, which was painful. I have spent many hours, and dollars, getting professional help. It was well worth the time, cost, and effort to learn to have mental health.

Health History

The information sheet below would have helped my doctor when I was manic in 2007. I had been stable for the ten or so years that I had been his patient. He had not seen me manic before. Plus, he did not know what medications or their dosages I had been on before becoming his patient. After I was stable again, we created this list of what would have helped him in giving me medication. I had a copy of my past medical records and created a list of medications I had tried from my medical records. I remembered some of the dosages and side effects but not all them. I recommend anyone on medication for any reason to keep a list like this. It is very valuable for your doctor and, in the long run, for you and your health. I gave the list of medication and dosages to my doctor, who put it into the computer for later use.

My Treatment History

Date: _____
Medication prescribed:_____
Dosage: _____
How often and when do I take it? _____
Side effects I have had: _____
Does it help me? _____

My Best Hospital Experience

My best hospital experience took place at Telecare Heritage Psychiatric Health Center in Oakland, California. I was hospitalized twice there in 2011 because I was classified as "gravely disabled." The only other classifications for being hospitalized are "a threat to yourself or someone else." My psychologist at Kaiser bipolar support group said they only classify homeless people as "gravely disabled." Since I was taking care of my finances, cooking for myself, cleaning my house, etc., he said I should not have been hospitalized. However, my family thought I should be because I was so manic.

The staff, except for one psychiatrist, was wonderful. That one psychiatrist, whom I happened to have, was a problem for many of the patients, not only me. To describe the doctor might be the best way for you to understand him. This is how people are medicated incorrectly. He wore a suit with a stiff white shirt, a tie, and boots. He appeared void of personality. His office was bare, except for his huge binders that were for each patient. The binders were the way the staff kept track of each patient. One time this doctor told me that I was "too happy and needed to have more medication." The other staff tried their best to make the patients comfortable, educated, and happy. This psychiatrist put me on Haldol, which is a very old drug. He put me on Benadryl so I could sleep, plus Valproic Acid in liquid form. I had been taking Valproic Acid in capsule form for years. Benadryl might help other people to sleep but not for me, especially when I am manic. Yet I could not sleep because of my roommate talking in her sleep and snoring. This doctor would not let me go home until I could sleep all night. As a result of the lack of good medication, I spent more time in the hospital but was still manic when I went home anyway.

The other doctor that I finally had enough nerve to request was great. This office was full of plants, pictures, and a rocking chair. It even had a boat made out of wood that the psychiatrist had made, and yes, he had those big binders. He also had access to all my medical records, which the first psychiatrist did not have. He, at least, let me go home. If I had had him earlier in my stay, the medication might have been different.

I know from experience that the mental hospitals, jails, and prisons do not get the newer drugs. This is because of the expensive cost. The second doctor might have changed my medication sooner. Yet before I left the hospital, I had an appointment with my regular Kaiser psychiatrist. I also had an appointment for the Kaiser Intensive Outpatient Program (IOP). The IOP is a class that was three days a week to keep people out of the hospital. It is also for a program for after the hospitalization, which is why I was taking it.

At Telecare, there was outside time two times per day. There was basketball, Frisbee, and two cats to pet. They had yoga mats to lay on the grass, and even apple and lemon trees with fruit that we could pick. When we were not able to go outside, there were beautiful outdoor pictures on the walls in the hall. I used these pictures to imagine being outside. They had games to play, TV, headset for music, and classes to attend. They had a musician that played a wonderful guitar and had great songbooks with music from the fifties and sixties to sing. They showed movies at night. The food was great with three meals a day and snack time. The staff did a daily check in for both staff and patients for a chance to talk about our feelings and anything bothering us. They encouraged us to check in. The staff was always interested in how to make our stay more comfortable and to change for the better. My suggestion to make this an ideal hospital would be to have private rooms, plus the use of modern medicine, both of which are expensive. I also suggested they get new basketballs (the old ones were flat). I wore my regular clothes. They had a washer and dryer where I could wash them. When they were in the wash, I borrowed the hospital's cloth gowns and pants. The gowns were typical hospital gowns, open in the back. I wore two gowns, one on backward. The site itself was pleasant with a creek outside. Unfortunately, we could not get to it because we were locked in but we could look at through the big windows. In the dining room (two stories high), there was a huge mural of a waterfall.

I was there for a purpose, if only to be writing about it to help other people. I miss the friendly and caring staff, but I do not miss the experience of being in lockup. I still am doing all I can to stay out of the hospital. Besides the experience of having a bad psychiatrist, I had very few visitors. This was because of the distance from my home. Yet I did have use of the phone, which was second best to having visitors.

My worst experience at Telecare, besides flat basketballs, was the pens we had to write with. They were not pens, but pen refills without the pen itself. I tried to write my bubble technique, which was difficult to do. Even in jail they give you real pens!

Compare the above to my worst hospital experience where I was in lockup five days at a local hospital. The only thing I could do in five days was to go on a picnic at a local lake. At the hospital, the only activity I had was pacing the halls. I could not read the magazines that my family brought for me because the medication made my eyes blurry. There was a TV that another patient controlled. There was a fenced-in yard. But no one could go outside because of staff shortage or they did not have time to watch everyone or just did not want to bother. There were no stall doors in the bathroom, and there were feces on the bathroom floor. No one encouraged me to bathe, so I was not aware I needed to for several days. I wore my own clothes for the entire five days. They did not have a washer and dryer. Thank goodness the county closed this hospital. The advantage of the local hospital was being allowed to have visitors. Yet my daughter should not have come to visit because she was underage (she was fourteen at the time). But she was tall, did not look her age, and slipped through. The only thing I was grateful for was the psych tech on staff. She was a former friend from high school about four hundred miles away. Since then, we have gotten together for many lunches.

Self-Rating Mood Scale		
10	Elated, raging, incoherent, belligerent, can't stop talking, overactive, not sleeping at all, hallucinating, paranoid	Needs hospitalization
Manic		
9	Elated, can't rate self, delusion of grandeur, belligerent, distortion of time, disdainful, unable to control emotions or thoughts	Needs more or different medication
8	Feel everything is working perfect, elated, sleeping very little, hostile when crossed, racing thoughts, inappropriate spending	Needs medication
Hypomanic		
7	Overactive, overly talkative, many ideas for new projects, scattered creativity, socially inappropriate, sleeping 4–6 hours, feels wonderful, mildly obtrusive	Check medication

6	Normal, feel positive, confident, creative, high energy, perceptive, confident, awareness of hyperactivity, may want to spend money and travel	
5	Normal, feel good, productive, good concentration, takes one day at a time, deal with problems as they arise. Can plan ahead and carry through, sense of balance	
4	Normal, mild depression, lack of energy, feels slowed down, anxiety, decreased motivation, going through the paces	
3	Moderate depression, loss of energy, disinterest in others, weight, sleep and appetite disturbances, function with effort, lot of anxiety, feel life not worthwhile, isolated	
Depressed		
2	Depressed, feel abandoned, serious sleep disturbances, very withdrawn, suicidal ideation, not acts, obsessing thoughts	Call doctor, call support group

1	Very depressed, withdrawn, extremely agitated or catatonic, difficulty rating self, suicidal	Needs hospitalization
Severely Depressed		
0	Unable to eat or take medication, can't follow routine, delusional, stuporous, stares into space, very little response when questioned	Needs medical help

Note: Developed by the leader of a Depressive (Uni polar) and Manic Depressive (Bipolar) self-help group at Herrick Hospital in Berkeley, California.

I want to comment on the self-rating mood scale. Number 7 says if you get four to six hours of sleep to check your medication. You are in a hypomanic state and risk getting manic. For years I figured if I got eight hours of sleep, I was doing well. Even my doctors thought eight hours was plenty of sleep for me. Yet I kept getting manic and was put in the hospital. I was following this chart, so I could not understand why I was still having trouble with the mania. Then I realized that I had to adjust my chart to fit me and my sleep habits. If I get four to six hours of sleep over several days or weeks, **I am manic** and need to be in the hospital. Now if I get nine to ten hours of sleep, I have to check my medication. My normal amount of required sleep is twelve to thirteen hours per night, sometimes even more. I remembered when I was a child and a young adult, I got teased because I slept too much. Now that I know twelve to thirteen hours the normal for my body, I hope I can stay out of the hospital! Only time will tell. The other thing that I have worked hard on is lowering my stress level. With the combination of sleep and lowered stress level, I can remain stable.

Personal Experiences

My Story: Part C

Do you know how to recognize, cope, and get relief from your emotions? After all, we all have emotions and feelings. They are what make us tick. In working with people in the past, I have found that someone has to be in bad shape to **want** to change their behavior. My main question to people is, "Is there something about yourself that you do not like. Is there something that you wish you could change?" If so, **you can change**. How do I know this? It is because I have changed. But it has taken many years of hard work to do these changes. I have had help from others too. I have had help from twelve step programs. Self-help books, the Psalms, psychologists, and therapists have helped. I have also had help from support groups and psychiatrists. Even my regular doctor, friends, and family have helped. I have learned from my worst as well as my best experiences.

I was too miserable not to change because of my life circumstances and because I did not like myself the way I was. I was miserable and did not have peace of mind. I am grateful that I have changed because I am much happier and more at peace. Am I where I want to be in life? No, I still am a work in progress, which I always hope to be, as long as I am alive. I do not want to have a stagnant life. I want to live my life to the fullest! Am I aware of my feelings? Yes, most of the time, which I was not able to do at all when I first started on my journey. Then there are the times that I fall back into old habits.

Life is full of hills and valleys, so I am sure that there will always be where I am not present and in control.

If you look on the following pages, you will notice my symptoms of when I am manic or depressed. Bipolar is only one of many diagnoses in categories of mental illness. But I am including a list of my symptoms. I am doing this to show what my family, friends, and I have to put up with when dealing with my bipolar disorder. This will help you identify the same in yourself, your family members, neighbors, or others. The mania has caused me the most trouble. When I am at my worst, I act like I am on crack cocaine. I get psychotic. People can get psychotic whether or not they have bipolar. Not getting enough sleep or being on drugs can cause psychosis. When I get psychotic, it is like I am dreaming. I do not see or hear anything and have no control over what I say or do. In my case, it is because my brain chemistry is going haywire. It is not doing what it is supposed to do or my medication stops working. At that point, I have no judgment or concentration or control.

Some things I remember doing, and some I do not, but I hear about them later from people who have observed and told me.

After I am hospitalized, it is like going through major surgery. It takes time, sometimes weeks or months, to rest and relax, to recuperate. Getting back into my normal routine helps me heal.

My Symptoms and Side Effects

When I am depressed, I forget to eat and/or do not want to eat and/or overeat, do not shower, cannot get out of bed, feel isolated and lonely, have a very low energy level, have suicidal thoughts and have had a plan, do not cook, have trouble concentrating and remembering things, have difficulty making decisions, have trouble getting to sleep but then sleep too much, have no sexual desire, feel hopeless and pessimistic and have the feeling that no one is there for me, worry and have anxiety about everything, feel ashamed about having a mental illness, feel worthless and unimportant, feel antisocial and standoffish, cry inappropriately, do not feel like doing anything, fear losing my mind and being out of control and being admitted to the hospital, have upset stomach and muscle aches when anxious, and hide my anger and other feelings. This list can be a useful list to check to see if you are depressed. If you have only a few depressive symptoms, you should also tell your health- care provider. Sometimes, a few symptoms can go on to become major depressive disorder. Some forms of depression are mild. But if symptoms are persistent or chronic, you may need treatment by a professional.

When I am manic, I have racing thoughts (my body is restless) and cannot sleep (and my medication stops working); forget to eat; have shallow breathing; make a lot of mistakes, do not cook (too busy with thoughts) and forget about food or eating; cannot concentrate on important things (too busy with my thoughts); talk loud and fast and inappropriate; have religious grandiosity; cannot follow a conversation, which makes it hard to follow instructions; am preoccupied and worried about the future and not living in the moment; have grand illusions about world peace; can do no wrong and know everything; am unable to focus when driving, therefore should not be driving; see great significance to all my writing, reading, what's on TV, radio, and what people say and want to share that with the world; want a tape recorder for my brain and my great thoughts; write compulsively and am compulsive about making lists; while trying to have a conversation, change the subject to my agenda and am forceful in doing so; act inappropriately, including sexually (according to my own standards); make wild plans and expect others to go along with me; am belligerent; ran naked in the neighborhood; pull out the mailbox post; destroy things in the house; give away possessions; put jewelry all over the house in sets of three items; cannot type as usual; and have papers all over my desk.

If you have had four of these symptoms at one time for at least one week, you may have had a manic episode. Tell your health-care provider about the episode. There are effective treatments for this form of bipolar.

My Side Effects from Psychiatric Medications

1. Full body rash
2. Dizziness
3. Flat affect / loss of personality
4. Severe tremors
5. Swelling of the feet four times in size

6. Diarrhea
7. Nausea
8. Weight gain*
9. Headaches
10. Tingling of the mouth
11. Feeling dazed
12. Restless leg syndrome
13. Hair loss
14. Occasional extreme fatigue
15. Slurred speech
16. Dry mouth
17. Bloody nose
18. Wobbly when getting up
19. Drowsy
20. Difficulty concentrating
21. Blurred vision
22. Sinus drainage
23. Lack of sexual desire*
24. Swelling of the feet, have to wear compression hose*
25. Low white blood cell count
26. Occasional shaky hands
27. Occasional drippy nose*
28. Sleep a lot
29. Severe constipation

* Current side effects

I list the above side effects to show that it is possible to have side effects from medication. Then go on and try other medications that might work better. Many people will not try a new medication for fear of the side effects.

Do not let your fear get the best of you. Still, pay attention to the side effects and only put up with the ones that you can tolerate. Consider which is the worst, your illness and symptoms or the side effects. If the side effects are not tolerable, ask your doctor to give you something else or try a different dose. Can you learn from my experiences, even if you do not have bipolar? You bet! Ask yourself if you are happy with your life and your relationships. Have you ever had thoughts racing around and around in your head, plus worrying about something so much you cannot sleep? If so, you can learn something from reading the **Tools for Stability** and working on yourself.

My Story: Part D

I hesitate to write my worst experiences, because I have worked so hard to put them in the past and stay in the present. The other reason I hesitate to write them is it is painful for my family and friends to rehash that pain. But it is much better for everyone to talk, read, or write about the "elephant in the room." This is a phrase I learned about in twelve-step programs. I can do nothing to change the past or the future for that matter. I can only learn from the past and can only change the present, the only minute I have to change. I know what I have gone through seems like nothing to what some others have been through in their lives. Yet, by you knowing what I have been through and overcome, it will give you hope that you too can overcome your issues. I want you to know that all my days are not perfect. Sometimes, I have difficulty staying in the present and having peace of mind. So, my mental health is my number 1 priority for every day.

So here is my list of trials that I have been through (besides having the mental illness diagnosis of bipolar: I have experienced low self-esteem, being a poor student until I left high school. (I made the dean's list for the first time when I was forty-eight years old!) I have gone through a messy divorce. I have dealt with the death of friends and family, plus extended family members who have committed suicide, and having had suicidal thoughts myself. I was asked to leave more than one job. I lost another job because the office closed and I did not want to move to Fresno to keep it. I did not have enough money to buy healthy food. I have had to sell my home because I could not afford to fix it. I have lived in an abusive relationship and living with addictions. The worst was PTSD from being molested as a child, which I wrote about earlier.

Most people who know me do not know that when I was in my twenties, I was afraid to go outside by myself. I only went out of the house when I was with a family member or friend. I hid behind my sunglasses, thinking people could not see me. It has taken many years to feel comfortable in public. In spite of my wanting to hide, I always had a smile on my face so no one would know I was afraid. Now I can even go on vacation by myself! Yet there are still things that I am uncomfortable with, like eating in a restaurant by myself when I travel alone, which is something I have to force myself to do. I have been practicing eating in a restaurant alone. It is getting more comfortable. Yet it depends on the restaurant. If it is fast food, I am okay, but a fancy restaurant is still uncomfortable eating alone. It is too bad I do not live in Europe where I could walk up to a table of people and ask if I could join them. This is my next step. I should start doing here in my own hometown, and start a new fad! To overcome being afraid, I have had to force myself to change, which was very difficult to do. Then again, I was so uncomfortable I had the desire to change myself.

In my twenties, along with being afraid to go out by myself, I was so depressed that I could not take care of my two children like a healthy mom should. I also could not do my household chores. My husband at the time was working full time and going to school full time, so he was not aware of my emotional state. Or if he was aware, he did not suggest that I get help, nor could we have afforded it, if he had. This was before I knew of 12-Step programs. If I had gone to 12-Step program maybe it would have helped my relationship with my husband. I often wonder what our lives would have been like had I changed at that time. Yet that was not my purpose in life. My purpose was to go through more trials in order for you to read the Tools for Stability and my life experiences.

If you are unaware of your feelings, you are stuffing them, like I used to do. Now I do not stuff my feelings as much as I used to, but I still catch myself in the "no feelings mode." If you journal about what feelings you recognize, it will help you.

Picture a page full of faces with different expressions that go with feelings. My challenge to you is to see if you can recognize your feelings with faces. Here are some suggested feelings to use: Aggressive, angry, anxious, ashamed, bashful, and bored. Cautious, confident, confused, curious, depressed, determined, and disappointed. Disbelieving, disgusted, ecstatic, embarrassed, enraged, envious, and exasperated. Exhausted, frightened, frustrated, grieved, and guilty. Happy, hopeful, hurt, indifferent, and interested. Jealous, joyful, lonely, loved, loving, or miserable. Optimistic overwhelmed, pained, puzzled, and regretful. Relieved, sad, satisfied, shocked, and shy. Smug, sorry, stubborn, stupid, surprised, suspicious, thoughtful, and withdrawn.

See if you can think up some more feelings and/or draw faces. Use your journal to draw your faces with different feelings.

Once you figure out your feelings, the following helps. At least it helped me.

The following list is from the Bible given to me by a friend. I was not much of a Bible reader at that time, so I was not sure they would help me, but they did. I would figure out how I was feeling or what I wanted and look up which psalm would help me. Some helped more than others. I include them in my book because I decided to include everything that helped me get better. I am not suggesting you use them if you are not a Bible reader. That is your choice. I am sharing what helped me.

Where to Find Help in the Book of Psalms

When you feel
  Afraid: vs. 3, 4, 27, 46, 49, 56, 91, 118
  Alone: vs. 9, 10, 12, 13, 27, 40, 43

Burned-out: vs. 6, 63
Cheated: vs. 41
Confused: vs. 10, 12, 73
Depressed: vs. 27, 34, 42, 43, 88, 143
Distressed: vs. 13, 25, 31, 40, 107
Elated: vs. 19, 96
Guilty: vs. 19, 32, 38, 51
Hateful: vs. 11
Impatient: vs. 13, 27, 37, 40
Insecure: vs. 3, 5, 12, 91
Insulted: vs. 41, 70
Jealous: vs. 37
Like quitting: vs. 29, 43, 145
Lost: vs. 23, 139
Overwhelmed: vs. 25, 69, 142
Penitent/sorry: vs. 32, 51, 66
Proud: vs. 14, 30, 49
Purposeless: vs. 14, 25, 39, 49, 90
Sad: vs. 13
Self-confidence: vs. 24
Tense: vs. 4
Thankful: vs. 118, 136, 138
Threatened: vs. 3, 11, 17
Tired/weak: vs. 6, 13, 18, 28, 29, 40, 86
Trapped: vs. 7, 17, 42, 88, 142
Unimportant: vs. 8, 90, 139
Vengeful: vs. 3, 7, 109
Worried: vs. 37
Worshipful: vs. 8, 19, 27, 29, 150

When you want
- Acceptance: vs. 139
- Answers: vs. 4, 17
- Confidence: vs. 46, 71
- Courage: vs. 11, 42
- Fellowship with God: vs. 5, 16, 25, 27, 37, 133
- Forgiveness: vs. 32, 38, 40, 51, 69, 86, 103, 130
- Friendship: vs. 16
- Godliness: vs. 15, 25
- Guidance: vs. 1, 5, 15, 19, 25, 32, 48
- Healing: vs. 6, 41
- Hope: vs. 16, 17, 18, 23, 27
- Humility: vs. 19, 147
- Illumination: vs. 19
- Integrity: vs. 24, 25
- Joy: vs. 9, 16, 28, 126
- Justice: vs. 2, 7, 14, 26, 37, 49, 58, 82
- Knowledge: vs. 2, 8, 18, 19, 25, 29, 97, 103
- Leadership: vs. 72
- Miracles: vs. 60, 111
- Money: vs. 15, 16, 17, 49
- Peace: vs. 3, 4
- Perspective: vs. 2, 11
- Prayer: vs. 5, 17, 27, 61
- Protection: vs. 3, 4, 7, 16, 17, 18, 23, 27, 31, 91, 121, 125
- Provision: vs. 23
- Rest: vs. 23, 27
- Salvation: vs. 26, 37, 49, 126
- Stability: vs. 11, 33, 46
- Vindication: vs. 9, 14, 28, 35, 109

Wisdom: vs. 16, 19, 64, 111

When you're facing
    Atheists: vs. 10, 14, 19, 52, 53, 115
    Competition: vs. 133
    Criticism: vs. 35, 56, 120
    Danger: vs. 11
    Death: vs. 6, 71, 90
    Decisions: vs. 1, 119
    Discrimination: vs. 54
    Doubts: vs. 34, 37, 94
    Evil people: vs. 19, 35, 36, 49, 52, 109, 140
    Enemies: vs. 3, 25, 35, 41, 56, 59
    Heresy: vs. 14
    Hypocrisy: vs. 26, 28, 40, 50
    Illness: vs. 6, 139
    Lies: vs. 5, 12, 120
    Old age: vs. 71, 92
    Persecution: vs. 1, 37, 56
    Poverty: vs. 9, 10, 12
    Punishment: vs. 6, 38, 39
    Slander/Insults: vs. 7, 15, 35, 43, 120
    Slaughter: vs. 6, 46, 83
    Sorrow: vs. 23, 34
    Success: vs. 18, 112, 127, 128
    Temptation: vs. 38, 141
    Troubles: vs. 32, 55, 86, 102, 142, 145
    Verbal cruelty: vs. 35, 120

In the World

My Story: Part E

What I have learned are little lessons that have helped me live my life so I had peace of mind, even in a world of turmoil. The only way I can live with peace of mind is to know I can change only myself and no one else. Nor can I change anything going on in the world.

You too cannot change anyone else, only yourself. With lots of work, you too can change to have peace of mind. That peace can radiate out into your relationships and your community. It takes baby steps, sometimes even one step forward and two steps backward.

My biggest help has been my faith, which was nonexistent before May 11, 1987, even though I went to church. That day was the first day I was locked in the hospital. This was after a sleepless weekend of compulsive writing, plus having to have someone tell me to eat. God told me I was his voice. Doctors have said I was hearing voices. When I have told this to other people over the years, they do not believe me but I do not care what they believe. No matter what, that experience has changed my life forever.

I was now starting a long twelve-year journey to get good quality medical care by a psychiatrist. Many people do not have to wait that long to get quality medical care. The good thing that has come of this entire long journey is being allowed to create and write my book. Plus, having my mental health as good as it is. Does this mean I am through learning? No! But I am changing and taking baby steps, because that is life.

Over the years, my faith has grown as I have changed. Because I do not want to step on anyone's toes, I try very hard to live my faith but not to preach it. Anyone is free to believe or not to believe. The most important thing is how we treat others. Yet I know for myself that I doubt I would be here without my faith in my God. When I am scared, I pray and imagine I am in a protective bubble. Nothing can hurt me. That has helped me get through my personal hell. This is how I managed to get out in public places and not be afraid anymore.

Volunteering and Employment - Benefits and Barriers

People with low self-esteem or disabilities have barriers to volunteering and employment. Yet these can be overcome. Your life can change for the better. With small steps, you can move forward.

By keeping an **"I can do it!"** attitude, you will find great possibilities.

Some of this came from the Sonoma County Volunteer Center.

Benefits of Volunteering or Working

Get your mind off your disability. There is more to life than your disability. This is the best advantage of working or volunteering. It can be very freeing to not feel that your disability is the most important thing in your life.

Gain self-esteem. Feeling useful brings happiness and positive things back into your life. **When we give, we get back.** We all have something to give.

Increase your income. Volunteering can sometimes lead to a paying job that allows you to live above the poverty line. Your wants, as well as your needs, can be met. Having a little bit more money still might not get you above the poverty line, but it can help anyway.

Gain experience. Learn new skills and add current experience to your resumé. These new skills and current resumé might lead to a better-paying or more rewarding job in the future.

Come out of isolation. Working develops communication skills. Getting out in the working world adds people and tasks to our lives, thus helping maintain mental health.

Give structure to your day. A regular schedule maintains mental health.

Take on more responsibility. Volunteering or working increases your self-esteem and fights depression.

Be useful and involved. Volunteering or working allows us to expand our sense of purpose. You are not in this world to exist. There is more to it than that. We are all valuable and have something to contribute. In this tough economy, even volunteers can be used more than ever to help make our world a better place.

You have a disability and want to work, but you can no longer work at your former job due to your disability. There is help to get retrained for a different kind of work. You can go to the State Department of Rehabilitation if you have a disability. They will give you ability tests and interview you for likes and dislikes. Plus, they will pay for you to get retrained. They will even pay for tools of your trade, like a special computer, phone, or other equipment. You can even start your own business. I know many people that are quadriplegic or paraplegic that work full time. Some of them have attendants or a service dog to help them. Goodwill Industries also helps with job training. I have had help from both of these agencies.

Do not give up on your dreams!

Barriers to Volunteering and Employment

"I can't" or *"I'm disabled"* or *"I'll get sick"*—these attitudes are the main barriers to volunteering or working. Changing these negative attitudes is possible but challenging. It is scary to get out there. To move beyond our fears takes constant reminders that *"I can do this!"* and *"I will do this!"* and *"Nothing will stop me from doing this or working!"* Many people have forgotten how to dream and hope. Acknowledge the fear and build on your hopes. If you have not done it before, volunteering can be hard but it is possible, one step at a time. The more you give, the more you will receive.

Fear of losing benefits from Social Security (SSDI) or Supplemental Security Income (SSI) can be scary. Both SSDI and SSI programs allow people to work and keep their medical benefits up to a certain income level. Learn how work will affect your disability benefits by consulting with one of Disability Services and Legal Center's Benefit Counselors or contact Social Security.

Fear of rent increase from HUD/Section 8 or other subsidized housing can come with making more money. Making more money will increase your rent, if you live in subsidized housing. Yet it might also allow you to live where you want to live. You will not have the financial restrictions you do when you live in subsidized housing. You won't have the dreaded housing inspections that you have with subsidized housing. This can be very freeing.

Stress causes symptoms for people with mental disabilities or those without a diagnosis. Plan to overcome the stress by building in support and taking small steps. Finding the right employer, hours, and type of work will help relieve stress. Volunteer someplace first to see if you like the people and atmosphere. Learn the job requirements and to find out how many hours you can work. Often employers would rather hire the volunteer they know than hire someone unknown. They will already know how you get along with the rest of their staff. Plus, they will know about your work ethics before spending a lot of time and money training you.

Fear of what people will think of you. It is safe at home. Overcoming the fears and getting out there anyway will give you a great sense of power. Make a pro and con list. What would be the very worst thing that would happen if you did volunteer or work? How would you deal with it? Is it any worse than the horror stories you have already dealt with in your life? Ask for support from a friend, family member, or support-group member. Try finding a job coach.

Goodwill has job coaches. Face your fears. Ask a friend or family member to do a "book end". This is where you call them before you try something. Then go do something you are afraid of and report back. Break things down into little doable pieces. Possible steps are phoning about the job and walking in the door to check the building out. Talking to someone there who is friendly. Volunteer for an hour a week and adding time as you feel comfortable. These steps will take months to do, but little steps can ease your fears. If you have a bad experience with a particular job, do not give up. Try another place or another type of job. If you feel uncomfortable working with people, try a job working with animals, plants, or trees. The more you do something, the less fearful you become.

The stigma of having a mental illness is one of the hardest things to overcome. Society makes people with mental illness know they are at the very bottom of the human scale. It takes time to realize and believe that having a mental disability is no big deal. You have to get your sleep and take your medication. You will learn to adjust like it is like having any other kind of disability. A mental disability is not a character defect! It's something that has gone wrong with your brain chemistry. That is why a mental disability is no different from a physical disability. Stand up for yourself. You are worth it! The best way to deal with stigma is to face it and set an example as someone who is dealing with their disability. When people get to know you, the more they will be able to understand plus accept you. To do this, you need to make your mental health your top priority. You can do this by learning and practicing staying stable. Most people who are stable now had failures along their way to stability. Even famous people have failures. It is part of living. Failing only means we get up, get going, and try again.

Lack of Experience Volunteering adds to your experiences, making it easier to get a paying job. As a volunteer, you have to be as responsible about your job as a paid person would. You have to be reliable, do the job, no matter how boring. Ask questions when you do not understand. Do the best job you can. Come to work as scheduled. Call in when you are not able to work, and get along with people—both coworkers and the public. You can list volunteer work as work experience on any résumé.

Loss of a sense of being useful causes a lot of depression and feelings of worthlessness. Helping other people with small jobs will increase your sense of self-worth. Start small! Find a person who needs help with yard work, cooking, shopping, or driving, etc. Volunteer to help them. Then branch out to something else. Keep adding to your résumé.

Lack of motivation stops a lot of people from moving forward. Go toward living a normal life of health, happiness, and well-being. No one can motivate you to do anything you do not want to do. Think of how your life is now. Are you miserable with the way things are? If so, give volunteering a try for a few months. Then check your life and see if you are feeling better. If you are, great! Keep up the good work. If you are not feeling better about yourself, switch to a different job to find a better fit. Give yourself another few months to see how it goes. If your volunteer job is going well, ask if you can work the volunteer job into a paying job.

Disclosure about your disability, whether it is physical or mental, is not required. That is unless you want a "reasonable accommodation" under the American Disability Act for your disability. For example, a reasonable accommodation might be shorter work hours. It might be longer breaks than other employees. Your disability is nobody's business but yours. Say you did not tell your employer about your disability, then after you started working you have symptoms that are causing you problems at work, your employer will have to know about your disability. My reasonable accommodation is shorter work hours during the week.

My Story: Part F

For almost 20 years I had an understanding employer. I had been in the hospital four times in those 20 years. Each time I have been in the hospital, I have missed work for at least a month. It takes a while to get back into working my normal schedule again. Even with my part-time schedule, I received earned time off that I could use for vacation or sick time. I still got paid. I have also at times used State Disability when I have been off work due to being manic. This has helped keep me from being homeless like many of the mentally ill people in our country.

I am fortunate in that I have worked the right amount of quarters to pay into Social Security in the past. So, I was receiving Social Security Disability Insurance (SSDI) for part of my income. This was because my disability would not allow me to work full time, take care of myself, and remain sane. Because I received SSDI, I also received Medicare to help me with my medical bills. Some people with a mental diagnosis or other disabilities are not able to work at all; some work full time. Now because I am over sixty-six years old, I receive a Social Security pension. Before I was sixty-six years old I had to report my income to Social Security and stay under SGA (Substantial Gainful Activity). I do not have to worry about my income amount any more.

Many people do not realize that Social Security is insurance that is part of the benefits of paying into it. This is from their paychecks. I paid in the past during my working career. In fact, Social Security and Medicare are still deducted from each of my paychecks. If I did not receive Social Security and I worked my regular part-time hours, I would not be able to pay my rent and other expenses. I would be homeless because I do not receive a high income. So, I receive both Social Security and work income. The two combined does not give me much money, but I have many blessings, which is worth more. Compared to the rest of the world, I am wealthy, as are most Americans.

Some people look down on people with disabilities as getting a free ride from the government. This is a huge sign of discrimination. They are confusing Social Security Disability Income (SSDI), which employees pay for, with Supplemental Security Income (SSI), which comes from taxes. Yet, even someone receiving SSI, which is for the disabled, should not be looked down on. I do not know anyone who wishes to be on SSI. This is with the exception of a disabled person with no income trying to qualify for SSI. Anyone can become disabled in a split second in a car accident or over a long period of time like me. SSI is for people who have never paid into Social Security and have a disability. A person does not qualify for SSDI if they did not pay into Social Security. This can include teachers, a person who has never worked, or someone who is self-employed. Many people on SSI, as well as many on SSDI, have to live below the poverty line! People on SSI are not allowed to have much money at all. Many people with disabilities work full time or part time. Some would love to work, but cannot find an employer that will hire them. This is because they have a disability. Even though it is against the law to discriminate against anyone who has a disability, employers find ways around the law all the time. Some people who have a disability are not able to work now. I encourage anyone with a disability to volunteer or work to help with their income as soon as they are able to do so. I also encourage people to change the law so those on disability do not have to live below the poverty level. Living below the poverty level is why we have so many homeless people with disabilities.

    Whether you have SSDI or SSI, if you want to work, you must find out as much information as you can before you go to work. This is to avoid an overpayment from Social Security.

Information List

Books, Organizations, Movies

The following are books, organizations, and movies are for widening your horizons. Some of them I have read and seen, and some, I have not. But they have chosen by others, so I have included them in the list. NAMI (National Alliance for the Mentally Ill; see **www.NAMI.org**) has a great library of books and movies. NAMI is a fantastic resource and support for family members. They have information, classes, and support for people with a mental illness diagnosis. They have offices all over the nation.

Books

The Language of Letting Go by Melodie Beattie
Believing in Myself by Earnie Larsen and Carol Hegarty
Alcoholics Anonymous Big Book from 12-Step Programs
Courage to Change from Al-Anon
Co-Dependent No More by Melodie Beattie
The Clutter Busting Handbook by Rita Emmett
Each Day a New Beginning by Hazelden Meditations
Pleasant Dreams by Amy Dean
Nourishing Traditions by Sally Fallon and Mary Enig, PhD
Moodswings by Ronald Fieve, MD
A Brilliant Madness by Patty Duke
Call Me Anna by Patty Duke
Touched by Fire: Manic Depressive Illness and the Artistic Temperament by Kay Redfield Jamison, PhD
Don't Sweat the Small Stuff for Teens by Richard Carlson
Life Strategies for Teens by Jay McGraw

Understanding Schizophrenia by Richard Keefe and Philip Harvey
The Power of the Other Hand by Lucia Capacchione, PhD
Wellness Recovery Plan by Mary Ann Copland
The Total Money Makeover by Dave Ramsey
Will I Ever Be Good Enough by Karyl McBride
14,000 Thing to be Happy About by Barbara Ann Kipfer
Helping Someone with Mental Illness: A Compassionate Guide for Family, Friends, and Caregivers by Rosalyn Carter with Susan K. Golant

Organizations in Sonoma County, California, and the Nation

Disability Services and Legal Center (707-528-2745) www.MyDSLC.org

Interlink Self-Help Center (707-546-4481) Santa Rosa www.interlinkselfhelpcenter.org

Wellness and Advocacy Center (707-565-7800) Santa Rosa www.wellnessandadvocacy.org

Russian River Empowerment Center (707-604-7264) Guerneville www.westcountyservices.org/pages/empowerment.html

NAMI (707-527-6655) Santa Rosa www.namisonomacounty.org

Sonoma County Mental Health (707-565-4850) www.sonoma-county.org

Alcoholic Anonymous www.sonomacountyaa.org

Narcotics Anonymous www.sonomacountyna.org

Innovations Community Center (707-259-8692) Napa www.innovationscommunitycenter.org

Depression Bipolar Support Alliance (800-826-3632) www.dbsalliance.org

National Schizophrenic Association (800-482-9534) www.sanonymous.org

National Mental Health Association (800-969-6642) www.nmha.org

National Psychiatric Association (888-357-7924) www.psych.org

Center for Journal Therapy (303-986-6460) www.journaltherapy.com

California Network of Mental Health Clients (800-626-7447) or www.californiaclients.org

St. Joseph's Behavioral Health (707-547-5450) www.stjosephhealth.org

Manzanita Services (707-463-0400) www.manzanitaservices.org

Department of Rehabilitation www.rehab.cahwnet.gov

Sonoma County Job Link (707-565-5550) www.sonomawib.org

Verity, Rape Crisis and Trauma Center (707-545-7273) www.ourverity.org

If you do not live in Sonoma County you can contact your local county Mental Health Department. Find out their organizations that help people with mental disabilities and their families.

Movies

Walking Across Egypt
Lars and the Real Girl
A Beautiful Mind
What About Bob
Patch Adams
Radio
Shine
Elling
Out of the Shadows
As Good As It Gets
Groundhog Day
What the Bleep Do We Know?
Michael Clayton
Mr. Jones
Silver Linings
Playbook
Frankie and Alice
One Flew over the Cuckoo's Nest

I do not know when I saw *One Flew over the Cuckoo's Nest* the first time. But it was before I was in the hospital in 1987. The very first time I received medication in the hospital, I thought of this movie. I do not know why I thought of it at that time. It was where Jack Nicholson pretended to take his medication. When given my medication at this hospital, I had to walk up to a window. They handed me my medication in a little white paper cup. They did not tell me what it was or the side effects. I did not want to take it. I did like Jack did and pretended to take my medication then threw the little cup and pill in the trash. No one knew I did not take my medication—that I know of. Later on, I must have caused trouble because when I became aware of where I was, there was a staff person between me and a man. I thought the man was my friend's dead husband and I needed to take him to her because she missed him so much. I do not know what I was doing to him, but it must have been serious enough to have a staff person there. The staff got me away from him. Then I saw a woman smoking by the staff desk, which it was okay to do at that time. I commented that she should not be smoking, which in my normal state I would not do. After that, about five staff members tackled me, gave me a shot, and put me in solitary confinement for the night. That was the first time of being in solitary. I do not remember much, but I stayed there all night long. Hollywood has a great effect on all, whether we are sane or not.

Conclusion

Melva Freeman

My Story: Part G

After my family left and after my divorce, I tried maintaining part ownership of my home. My former husband still owned part of the house. At that time, I was working full time but did not make enough money to do the repairs needed. Because my home was a fixer-upper, my therapist suggested I have roommates, even though I did not want to. The only reason I did was because I wanted to keep our house, thinking my husband would come back. Then we could finish fixing it up. Our house was a money pit with a fantastic view of the city. I did not realize how much of a money pit until I finally decided to sell it after my former husband remarried. I lived with roommates at my house for six years before finally deciding to sell it. It took two years to sell, and by then I was down to only one roommate. By then I had lost my full-time job. We decided that we could not afford to live alone, thus decided to still rent together to have lower rent. He was my last roommate, and I lived with him for eighteen years. We got along well, even though our lifestyles were different. We did not have a romantic relationship. He put up with my illness, even through four hospitalizations! Having him as a roommate allowed me to live where I could have all my belongings. Our duplex had a two-car garage, a yard, and I could have my own washer and dryer, plus it was in a nice neighborhood. We each had our own bedroom and bath. We even had a landlord that kept our rent reasonable so we could stay there. It too was a fixer-upper, but did not need as much fixing as my house did. Our landlord did some of the repairs, and so did we with her approval.

Having a roommate and being able to work allowed me some financial freedom. I have worked with many homeless people that would rather be on the streets than live with a roommate. This was because of bad experiences with roommates in the past or horror stories they had heard. I too have had bad experiences. But if you want to live someplace, you might have to make sacrifices work together to make it work. The best combination is someone you already know and like. Yet, even then, there can be conflicts. My roommate and I had met at a twelve-step group, but we did not know each other very well. We had mutual friends that thought we would make good roommates. First, you have to learn how to be at peace with yourself, then it will be easier to work with someone else. Learning the **Tools for Stability** can help in any type of relationship, not only helping to live and have peace of mind. Learning to express yourself in a nonthreatening way helps. Being respectful is most important. Even having house rules made up by the two of us helped. For example, making sure the dishes were clean after each meal. The main living areas were clean helped our relationship stay on an even keel. Since we each had our own bedroom and bathroom, we decided we each could keep our rooms as filthy or clean as we wanted.

My roommate and I had to leave our rental. We lived there for sixteen years. The owner was moving in. We decided to live apart because we each had separate dreams of where we wanted to live. By now I had learned enough about low-income housing that I was hoping I could find something. I was very fortunate that I found a wonderful apartment for seniors. It was well kept and beautiful (not the fixer-upper!). Most important it was quiet and had lots of activities and friendly people. My roommate found a cottage in the country that he could fix up with rent he could afford. I decided I like fixing things and doing construction. But after living in fixer- uppers most of my adult life, I was ready to live someplace nice. I can always help one of my kids or Habitat for Humanity, if I get the urge to fix something. It was a blessing that we were asked to move out of the duplex, because it burned down in the Santa Rosa fires in 2017. In 2019 fires in Geyersville the fires came within 10 feet of my former roommate's cottage.

To move and find an affordable apartment, I had to give up my garage, washer, and dryer. Plus, I had to get rid of a lot of treasures that I have enjoyed over the years. For years I had thought of things I would get rid of because I would have to move to a smaller place. I was grateful that the stress of moving did not make me manic or land me in the hospital again! I think that was because I was prepared to move someday. I am very fortunate to have found an apartment that I could afford and help from my children to move. I was lucky to find a tax credit low income apartment. So, my apartment is affordable and I have the advantage that if anything needs fixing all I have to do is fill out a request for repair form and it gets fixed.

Do I try and avoid getting manic? Yes, I do everything I can! Do I have any control whether I get manic? Yes and no. I have a brain chemistry problem that affects my moods sometimes. I have learned to say no when I am under too much stress so I can get my sleep, which is most valuable to my mental health. Am I always successful? No, sometimes I still get manic because that is the way my brain works. Sometimes my medication works, and sometimes it does not. Do I like it or choose to have a mental diagnosis? No, but that is my life.

Yet, there is also the question: do I have bipolar, or was I under too much stress, which caused me not to sleep? One time I was in the hospital because I was psychotic. I was thinking of my grandmother, whom I missed. It was Christmastime, and I was thinking of the past sexual abuse and not sleeping because of all the stress at work. When I got to the hospital, they immediately changed my medication. I could not sleep. Thus, I was still manic. Remember, anyone can get psychotic without sleep.

My question to my doctor, "Am I suffering from post-traumatic stress disorder? Did that cause me to not sleep?" We discussed PTSD. My doctor told me they sometimes use high-blood-pressure medication for people with PTSD. This is because sometimes people with PTSD suffer from high blood pressure. But I have low blood pressure, so if I took this medication, it could kill me. Again, each person has a different experience with medication.

I now live alone in an apartment that feels like a luxury hotel that I can afford. My current position as a companion caregiver allows me to have less stress. My moods have been normal for a long time. I am fortunate that I can now tell when I am getting close to mania. I know I will not go off my medication, even though I am doing well, unless my doctor says I can.

The last time I got manic was in May 2017 after I was in a head-on collision. I had to go to the emergency room for some minor injuries. I did not get home until 10:30 p.m. I usually go to bed around 7:00 p.m. It was late and I hurt, so I did not get a good night's sleep for several nights. I was busy filling out paperwork from my accident. I started to get manic, which I recognized. I called my doctor, and she changed my medication. I was off work for a month. My adult children wanted me to go to Casa Rohnert Park, a six-bed locked facility in my home town. That way I could be under more care than I would be at home. They took me to the emergency room so I could be evaluated by a doctor. The doctor did not think I was bad enough to be hospitalized. My son did take away the keys to my new car for a month. I was very stressed out because I had many doctor appointments to get to. I had to ask neighbors to take me. I do not like losing my independence. But years earlier I had asked my children to take my car keys if I was manic. I was very grateful not to have to go to the hospital.

The next time I was close to being manic was when we had all the bad fires in Santa Rosa. It stressed me out. It was a scary time for a lot of people. Disability Services and Legal Center, where I worked at the time manned a table at the local Press Democrat newspaper office. There were lots of agencies, including FEMA. A lot of fire victims were able to get information and to get help. I was in a hypomanic state. When I am in that state, I am close to being manic, but can function. My coworkers would not let me help out at the newspaper office due to the stress. They could tell when I start to get manic, and they knew I was close. So, I worked at our office, which was down the street from the newspaper office. I did go with a coworker to the table we were occupying and gave away some of my books. I decided this was one way I could help. I would not have been able to work there even if I was not close to being manic due to the noise level. I also have hearing issues that would interfere with my ability to help anyone.

So, dear reader, if you learn one thing from my experience, it is worth all the suffering I have been through. You cannot change the entire world, but you can change yourself. I know that because I have changed myself, and if I can do it, **you can too!** My world around me might in trouble, but for the most part I have peace of mind. What I teach in the **Tools for Stability** can help anyone to improve their mental health and to have peace of mind.

I received an interesting poem from a friend on Facebook that fits me perfectly after all these years. I want to share this with you. Maybe after all the reading you have done about the **Tools for Stability** and my story, you will be helped too.

If you are depressed, you are living in the past. If you are anxious, you are living in the future. If you are at peace, you are living in the present. (Lao Tzu)

I can say for today I have peace of mind. My moods have been fairly stable. I have not had the urge to write since I finished writing the first edition of my book. This has been a true blessing!

My blessings might be different than yours. But hopefully, this information is still helpful for you. Remember, everyone has their own journey to follow.

A favorite poem of mine is a Cherokee legend. It has many titles "The Wolves Within" or "Two Wolves" or "Grandfather Tells."

> One evening, an elderly Cherokee brave told his grandson about a battle that goes on inside people.
>
> He said, "My son, the battle is between two wolves' inside us all. One is evil. It is anger, envy, jealousy, sorrow, regret, greed, arrogance, self-pity, guilt, resentment, inferiority, lies, false pride, superiority, and ego. The other is good. It is joy, peace, love, hope, serenity, humility, kindness, benevolence, empathy, generosity, truth, compassion, and faith."
>
> The grandson thought about it for a minute and then asked his grandfather, "Which wolf wins?"
>
> The old Cherokee simply replied, "The one that you feed."

No matter what the title or where it came from, this tale is a terrific way to let you know that we all have those inner problems to overcome. It depends on which way we want to go in our lives that makes the difference. Whatever your problems, goals, or dreams, you can change your life if you really want to, depending on which wolf you feed. *Go for it!*

Some pages that are in my book have come from sources I do not remember but have helped me! For example, the "Don't Ever Give Up Bird and the Frog." In my imagination, the bird is the bipolar and I am the frog. I will **not** let the bipolar get the best of me. This picture, along with poems and sayings, were on my refrigerator or bathroom mirror for a long time. It helped to remind me to keep focusing on the better. What demons does the bird represent to you? As I have grown in my recovery, my picture has changed. In my imagination, I, as the frog, am sitting next to the bird (the bipolar). I still will not ever give up. The bipolar and I coexist in peace.

As I finish this book, I hope you have been helped in many ways. Remember, it took me over twenty-five years to learn all that I have included. My main reason for writing is so it does not take you that long. Learn what you can and remember to take baby steps and make time for fun. **Peace be with you on your journey!**

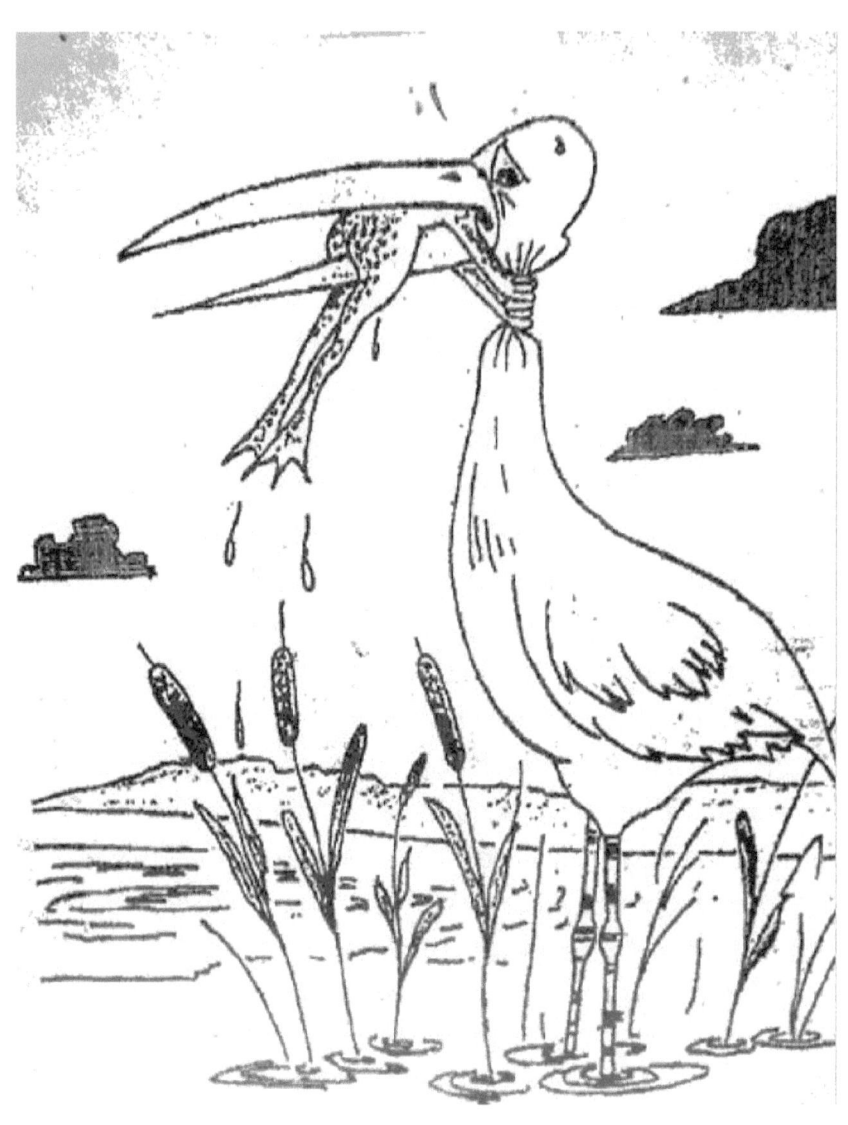

Don't EVER give up! ···

Acknowledgments

I appreciate all the trials and lessons I have learned from the medical community. That even includes doctors and psychiatrists that "did me wrong." It is my hope that they too can learn from reading the ***Tools for Stability*** book.

A special thank you to my former doctor, Virginia Hofmann, MD, for helping me with my medication to stay sane. And my current doctor, Jennifer Anne Cannon, MD for believing me when I told her I need medication help so I can make sure I get 12-13 hours of sleep per night to avoid getting manic.

Thank you to Mike Miller, MD, my former psychiatrist for over twelve years. He told me that my Tools for Stability would work for anyone, not only people with mental illness. Thanks for teaching me so much and making me feel okay with working part-time.

Thank you to Nick DeMara, PhD, and Sandra Seligson, PhD, at the Kaiser Permanente bipolar support group for their encouragement and words of wisdom.

Thank you to Mariah Day, MFCC, for teaching me boundaries, advising me to get roommates and helping me decide to sell my fixer-upper home that I could not afford.

Thank you to the pharmaceutical companies for making my medication that keeps me sane.

Thank you to my friends and family for putting up with my mania and psychosis, plus helping me when I needed to be in the hospital. Thank you for your visits to the hospital when I needed a familiar face. I especially want to thank my friends. They sent me cards of encouragement, special sayings, and poems. They fed me, clothed me, and entertained me. Thank you for doing the many activities with me and teaching me to do my finances. Thank you to my friend that helped me learn what to look for to find a compatible roommate.

Thank you to all the hospital staff for their lessons, both good and bad. Hopefully, someday our mental hospitals will be like the one I went to in Oakland, California. My hope is for people will get newer medication that works for them while they are in the hospital. Someday our prisons and jails will be for people who are criminals, not mental patients.

Thank you to Lt. Dave House from Sonoma County Main Adult Detention Center for taking the **Tools for Stability** workshop and introducing me to Lt. Corrado Ghioldi.

A special thank you to Lt. Corrado Ghioldi from the Sonoma County Main Adult Detention Center, Mental Health Unit, for giving me a tour of the jail and for giving me the honor of teaching the **Tools for Stability** workshop and my experiences as a mental patient to all his officers at the jail. Thank you for caring enough about your inmates to hire caring and empathetic officers for the mental health unit.

Thank you to my former employer, Disability Services and Legal Center. They allowed me to teach and write the **Tools for Stability** to use in our community. DSLC is a nonprofit organization that is classified as an independent-living center. Their mission statement is "Advancing the rights of people with disabilities to equal justice, access, opportunity, and participation in our communities."

Thank you to my publisher, Writers Branding for helping me publish my book so people can afford to buy it.

Thank you, dear reader, for reading this book. I hope it helped you from my experiences to overcome your own issues. I hope what I wrote helps you understand yourself and others.

Most of all, I thank my Creator who put the words at my fingertips, even compulsively in the middle of the night, and words in my mouth to help others.

My dream is for this book to go worldwide to as many people as possible.

About the Author

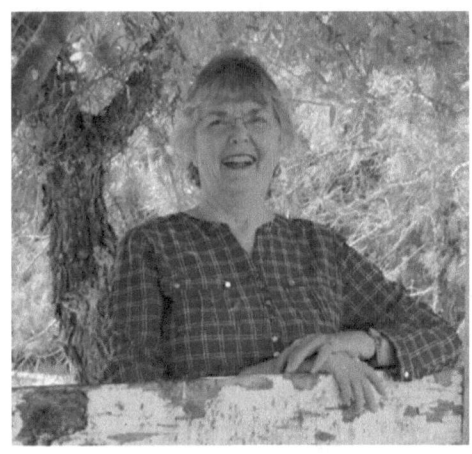

Melva Freeman started on the mental illness road in 1987 when she was thirty-nine years old. After she was misdiagnosed, she was finally diagnosed with bipolar disorder in 1990. Before her first hospitalization, she was married, with teenage children, active in her community (having 5 volunteer jobs), and worked parttime as a seamstress. After her first hospital experience, she went to work full time for an insurance company until the office closed. She was hospitalized again after her children left home. At one point, she found out that her symptoms were caused by stress and lack of sleep. This was told to her by friends in a support group who also said she was on too much medication not given by a psychiatrist. While going through a messy divorce, the empty-nest syndrome, having trouble finding and keeping work, and going to school part- time, Melva decided to go on disability. It took two years to qualify for, causing much financial hardship and stress. Melva ended up depressed, suicidal, and in bed most of the time. Melva has been involuntarily locked-in a mental hospital six times since 1987. Through this experience, she has gained knowledge to help others with a mental illness or a family or community member become healthier and happier.

www.ingramcontent.com/pod-product-compliance
Lightning Source LLC
LaVergne TN
LVHW040151080526
838202LV00042B/3111